Praise for
Mentoring Today's

"Who of us has not had a time when we needed some wise counsel? The Global Mentoring Process Model helps us see that what we do with each other can be done in different ways and yet contribute to the science of nursing. As this book points out, mentoring may occur at various levels throughout our lives, but the core is commitment to one another. Mentoring fills the gap of nuances, and specific advice is included in this book. Learning about being a professional without textbooks and lectures comes alive through experiencing how others are doing so. The final chapter, thoughts from Billye Brown and Sr. Rosemary Donley, provides sage advice about what it means to be a mentor—and to be mentored."

–Patricia S. Yoder-Wise, EdD, RN, NEA-BC, ANEF, FAAN
President, The Wise Group
Professor Emerita and Dean Emerita,
Texas Tech University Health Sciences Center School of Nursing

"Increasingly, nursing leaders are aware that we all function within a truly global village. This book offers numerous reality-based insights backed by existing scientific evidence that will prove beneficial for mentors as well as mentees at all educational levels, with consideration of the culture of organizations as well as the culture of ethnicity."

–Nancy C. Sharts-Hopko, PhD, RN, FAAN
Professor and Director, PhD Program
Villanova University College of Nursing

"The authors present a readable and carefully documented discussion and explanation of the critical role of mentorship in today's world of nursing. Identifying the issues that face contemporary nurses who aspire to leadership roles in international communities, the book provides practical guidance for implementing mentoring strategies in various health care settings and in multiple clinical, academic, research, and administrative roles. Practical advice is enhanced by personal reflections of current and past nurse leaders and mentors."

–Sr. Mary Jean Flaherty, PhD, RN, FAAN
Former Professor and Dean of Nursing at
The Catholic University of America

"The authors and contributors, well-known and respected mentors and protégés themselves, offer nurses in academic and health care settings a global and systems perspective of mentoring uniquely suited for today's health care environment. Drawing on their own experiences, the authors provide cultural understandings and advice about navigating complex systems for those entering into mentorship relationships; students in all types of academic programs, faculty, and practicing nurses worldwide will benefit from their wisdom. The TIPS (thoughts, ideas, possible strategies) provide practical advice for both mentors and mentees. The reflections about mentoring that punctuate this book will inspire the mentor within each of us."

–Diane M. Billings, EdD, RN, FAAN
Chancellor's Professor Emeritus
Indiana University School of Nursing

"Bond, Baxley, and Ibitayo not only know the nursing education culture, but they are passionate about mentoring as the method for equipping nurses for a global context. They do not rest on their past experiences but continue to grow as practitioners of mentoring. This book provides many practical tips and focused resources for the mentoring process."

–Linda Searby, PhD, Assistant Professor, Auburn University
–Mark Searby, DMin, Director of Doctoral Studies, Beeson Divinity School,
Samford University
Peacewood Consulting Services

"Mirroring challenges that face all nurses, these experienced authors offer practical, documented mentor-mentee strategies that foster intergenerational passing of the leadership torch. This unique approach offers their Global Mentoring Process Model, which is built upon a worldview of complexity theory and a systems thinking approach. As nurses progress in their careers and shift between new roles and new employment settings, they will find this book informative in shaping their connections and successful development as transformative leaders. Mentoring relationships are empowering, making the book a must-have for those who seriously entertain choosing or being mentor guides with each new career challenge."

–Cathleen M. Shultz, PhD, RN, FAAN, ANEF, CNE
Dean and Professor of Nursing
Harding University
Carr College of Nursing

"Mentoring nurses is an investment in the future of our profession. Mentors and protégés alike will find this book to be a valuable addition to their library, gleaning insight and wisdom from nursing leaders about the value of mentoring, regardless of career stage. A unique and important contribution of this book is its emphasis on the influence of culture in the mentoring relationship."

–*Judith A. Halstead, PhD, RN, ANEF, FAAN*
Professor of Nursing
Director, Office of Online Education
Indiana University

"Without a doubt, a must-have book on global mentoring. This book offers easy-to-read content and interpretation that allow the reader to gain an understanding of how valuable mentorship is for both the mentor and mentee."

–*Jose Alejandro, PhD, MBA, RN-BC, CCM, FACHE*
Executive Director of Case Management, Steward Health Care System
Former President, National Association of Hispanic Nurses
Treasurer, Case Management Society of America

Mentoring Today's Nurses
A Global Perspective for Success

Susan M. Baxley, PhD, RN
Kristina S. Ibitayo, PhD, RN
Mary Lou Bond, PhD, RN, CNE, ANEF, FAAN

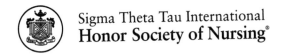

Sigma Theta Tau International
Honor Society of Nursing®

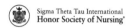
Sigma Theta Tau International
Honor Society of Nursing®

The Honor Society of Nursing, Sigma Theta Tau International (STTI) is a nonprofit organization whose mission is to support the learning, knowledge, and professional development of nurses committed to making a difference in health worldwide. Founded in 1922, STTI has 130,000 members in 86 countries. Members include practicing nurses, instructors, researchers, policymakers, entrepreneurs and others. STTI's 482 chapters are located at 626 institutions of higher education throughout Australia, Botswana, Brazil, Canada, Colombia, Ghana, Hong Kong, Japan, Kenya, Malawi, Mexico, the Netherlands, Pakistan, Portugal, Singapore, South Africa, South Korea, Swaziland, Sweden, Taiwan, Tanzania, United Kingdom, United States, and Wales. More information about STTI can be found online at www.nursingsociety.org.

Sigma Theta Tau International
550 West North Street
Indianapolis, IN, USA 46202

To order additional books, buy in bulk, or order for corporate use, contact Nursing Knowledge International at 888.NKI.4YOU (888.654.4968/U.S. and Canada) or +1.317.634.8171 (outside U.S. and Canada).

To request a review copy for course adoption, e-mail solutions@nursingknowledge.org or call 888. NKI.4YOU (888.654.4968/U.S. and Canada) or +1.317.634.8171 (outside U.S. and Canada).

To request author information, or for speaker or other media requests, contact Marketing of the Honor Society of Nursing, Sigma Theta Tau International at 888.634.7575 (U.S. and Canada) or +1.317.634.8171 (outside U.S. and Canada).

ISBN: 9781937554910
EPUB ISBN: 9781937554927
PDF ISBN: 9781937554934
MOBI ISBN: 9781937554941

Library of Congress Cataloging-in-Publication Data

Baxley, Susan M., 1946- author.
Mentoring today's nurses : a global perspective for success / Susan M. Baxley, Kristina S. Ibitayo, Mary Lou Bond.
   p. ; cm.
Includes bibliographical references and index.
ISBN 978-1-937554-91-0 (book : alk. paper) -- ISBN 978-1-937554-92-7 (EPUB) -- ISBN 978-1-937554-93-4 (PDF) -- ISBN 978-1-937554-94-1 (MOBI)
I. Ibitayo, Kristina S., 1964- author. II. Bond, Mary Lou, 1937- author. III. Sigma Theta Tau International, issuing body. IV. Title.
[DNLM: 1. Mentors. 2. Nursing--methods. 3. Nursing Methodology Research. 4. Nursing Staff--education. 5. Staff Development--methods. WY 18]
RT82
610.73--dc23
                    2013033002

First Printing, 2013

Publisher: Renee Wilmeth
Acquisitions Editor: Emily Hatch
Editorial Coordinator: Paula Jeffers
Cover Designer: Rebecca Batchelor
Interior Design/Layout: Katy Bodenmiller

Principal Book Editor: Carla Hall
Development and Project Editor: Brian Herrmann
Copy Editor: Heather Wilcox
Proofreader: Erin Geile
Indexer: Joy Dean Lee

Dedication

This book is dedicated to . . .

. . . my family and to my mentors along the way, but especially to Mary Lou, without whose mentoring this book would not be possible.

–Susan

. . . each mentor who walked with me in the various stages of my life, encouraging me, providing honest critique, and envisioning with me what was yet to come and how to reach my goals.

–Kristina

. . . all the global mentors who have provided me a guiding hand as I traversed the United States, Puerto Rico, and Mexico in my early nursing career and who continue to support me as I take on new initiatives.

–Mary Lou

Acknowledgments

The editors acknowledge the consistent assistance provided by individuals at the University of Texas at Arlington College of Nursing during the development of this book. Thank you for your commitment to helping us bring this project to completion. Specifically, we thank graduate research assistants Christy Bomer-Norton (RN, CNM, MSN, FBCLC), Whitney Mildren (RN, BSN), and Ignacio Godinez Puebla (MBA, MSc). Additional thanks go to Twanda Briggs (BS, AAAS), administrative services officer at the Center for Nursing Research.

We would also like to acknowledge our families and friends who have offered support and encouragement throughout the development of this book.

About the Authors

Susan M. Baxley, PhD, RN

Dr. Susan Baxley graduated with a bachelor of science in nursing from the University of Texas System School of Nursing. Her master of science is from Texas Woman's University, and her PhD is from the University of Texas at Arlington. During her education, she received scholarships and the Ferne and Evan Kyba dissertation fellowship to assist with her studies. She also received an award from Southern Nursing Research Society for the podcast *What Is a Nurse Scientist?* Baxley's research and publications have focused on Mexican women and mentoring.

Baxley has practiced nursing for more than 45 years, specializing in maternal-infant health. Her expertise in education and mentoring of patients, staff, and students led her to a research focus of women of Mexican origin becoming mothers. As a maternal-infant nurse with experience as an educator and program director, she has expertise in teaching and mentoring others by using special projects and creative program designs to achieve desired results. Baxley worked on several projects related to mentoring, including two research grants with a focus on the success of diverse students. As a clinical associate professor in the MSN program, teaching Research and Theory in Nursing, she mentors students in their understanding of the research process.

Baxley serves as director of the PhD in Nursing Mentoring Program, where she provides guidance and special programs for protégés and mentors that help the protégés become nurse scientists. This interest has led her to a new research focus on mentoring PhD students. She has served on the March of Dimes professional education committee in the Dallas/Ft. Worth, Texas area and currently serves on the Healthy Tarrant County Collaboration Steering Committee. She supports the university by serving on college of nursing and university committees. She also serves on dissertation committees and mentors honors students as they complete their theses.

Kristina S. Ibitayo, PhD, RN

Dr. Kristina Ibitayo is a graduate from Hesston College (ADN), and her education at the University of Texas at Tyler includes a bachelor of science in journalism, bachelor of science in nursing, master of science in nursing, and a master of science in human resource development. Her PhD in nursing is from the University of Texas at Arlington. She was recognized as a University Scholar and included in *Who's Who Among Students in American Colleges and Universities*. Scholarships and funding for her studies include the Mary Lou Bond dissertation fellowship.

Ibitayo has practiced nursing in a variety of settings and roles over the past 28 years. Her staff nurse experience includes medical/surgical, telemetry, emergency room, and perioperative nursing care. As a nurse manager, she oversaw the daily operation and performance improvement of four nursing units (Preadmissions, Same-Day Surgery, Post-Anesthesia Care Unit, and Pain Management). She was the system administrator for an operating room's specialized computer system and served as clinical support to the lead nurses. As a clinical assistant professor at the University of Texas at Arlington in the undergraduate nursing program, she annually mentors senior nursing students in their leadership/ management course and their capstone clinical experience.

Her nursing expertise and her childhood experiences in a rural clinic in Guatemala led her to pursue a PhD in nursing, with a research focus on internationally educated nurses (IENs) migrating to the United States. Ibitayo is one of the founders of the Good Seeds Ministry microenterprise lending program in Nigeria. Her professional service activities include conducting nursing seminars and workshops in Uganda and Rwanda with the North Texas Africa Health Initiative. She is also an educational associate for UT Arlington's Center for Hispanic Studies in Nursing and Health and has led students and health care professionals to Mexico for the center's Travel, Study, Learn program.

Ibitayo served as editorial assistant for the *Journal of Child and Adolescent Psychiatric Nursing*. She has presented her research at various nursing conferences, and she has extensively published her poetry in peer-reviewed nursing journals, nursing newsletters, brochures, and web pages. She has been invited to present her creative work at national conferences and used her poem "Doors of Opportunity" to guide her invited keynote address at Hesston College's pinning ceremony.

Mary Lou Bond, PhD, RN, CNE, ANEF, FAAN

Dr. Mary Lou Bond is a graduate of Bethel Deaconess Hospital (diploma), Texas Christian University (bachelor of science in nursing), the University of Pittsburgh (master of nursing), the University of Texas at Austin School of Nursing (PhD) and the School of Nurse Midwifery at El Centro Medico in Rio Piedras, Puerto Rico. She practiced nurse-midwifery in central Mexico before beginning her professional career as a faculty member, which has spanned teaching at all educational levels. As an educational administrator, she served as assistant dean and associate dean (University of Texas at Arlington College of Nursing [UTACON]) and as interim dean (University of Arkansas for Medical Sciences School of Nursing). She was the founding associate dean of the PhD in Nursing program at UTACON, which has had an active mentoring program for students since its inception.

Bond is assistant director of the Center for Hispanic Studies in Nursing and Health (CHSNH) and adjunct professor at UTACON. She was founder of the Challenge to Leadership Program, a forerunner of the UTA Hispanic Student Nurses' Association, and cofounder of the CHSNH (1996), which has the goal of fostering increased understanding between health providers and persons of Hispanic origin. She shared responsibility for the organization, implementation, and dissemination of proceedings from a series of International "Crossing Borders" conferences, and has organized and led numerous educational programs to Mexico for health care students and professionals. She has served on the Joint Commission on Accreditation of Hospitals and Organizations' Technical Advisory Panel on Culture, Language, and Health and the Board of Trustees for the Commission on Graduates of Foreign Nursing Schools (CGFNS). She was recently appointed to the roster of Fulbright Specialists.

Bond has received numerous awards, including the Lucy Harris Linn Excellence in Teaching Award and the Minority Health Nursing Research Award from the Southern Nursing Research Society. In 2010, she was selected as the outstanding alumna from the University of Pittsburgh

School of Nursing. She is an elected member of the American Academy of Nursing and the Academy of Nurse Educators of the National League for Nursing. Bond has published widely about issues related to barriers and supports for minority students, preparing nurses and nurse educators for work with Hispanic populations, and meeting tomorrow's health care needs through both local and global involvement.

Contributing Authors

Billye J. Brown, EdD, RN, FAAN

Billye J. Brown, dean of the University of Texas at Austin School of Nursing (UTA-SON) from 1972 until her retirement in 1989, has been working since then as an associate and consultant with Tuft & Associates, an executive search firm. She served as president of the American Association of Colleges of Nursing, the District Six Texas Nurses Association, and the Texas Nurses Association. She has served on numerous committees of the Texas Nurses Association, the American Nurses Association, the Texas League for Nursing, and the National League for Nursing. A fellow of the American Academy of Nursing, Brown was honored by that organization as a Living Legend in 2010. Long active in the Honor Society of Nursing, Sigma Theta Tau International (STTI), she served as the organization's president from 1989-91 and chaired or cochaired various committees, including the Project Advisory, Nominating, and Building Dedication Program committees. Brown received numerous awards over her long and distinguished career, including the Mary Tolle Wright Excellence in Leadership Founders Award (STTI, 1999); the Certificate of Distinction (Association of College Honor Societies, 2000); the Nell J. Watts Lifetime Achievement in Nursing Award (STTI, 2007); the Chapter's Mentor Award (Epsilon Theta Chapter of STTI, 1985); and Epsilon Theta Chapter, STTI Billye J. Brown Excellence in Leadership Award (2007). She served as an assistant editor of the *Journal of Professional Nursing* from 1985 to 1986. She is a member of the Chancellor's Council of the University of Texas System. In May 1991, the UTA-SON Alumni Association presented Brown with the Founders Award. In 1992, St. Joseph College awarded her an honorary Doctor of Humane Letters. Also in 1992, she was selected for the Hall of Fame, University of Texas School of Nursing at Galveston. Brown, a diploma graduate of the Arkansas Baptist Hospital School of Nursing, earned a bachelor's degree in nursing education from the University of Texas Medical Branch School of Nursing, a master's degree in nursing education from St. Louis University, and an doctor of education degree from Baylor University.

Paulette Burns, PhD, RN

Paulette Burns is dean of the Harris College of Nursing and Health Sciences at Texas Christian University (TCU) in Fort Worth, Texas. She holds a bachelor of science in nursing from the University of Maryland, a master of science with a clinical specialization in maternity nursing and nursing education from the University of Oklahoma, and a PhD in nursing from Texas Woman's University. Since beginning her nursing career 42 years ago in nursing staff positions in the U.S. Army Nurse Corps, her career has been in nursing education in faculty and higher education administrative roles. Her 24 years as an administrator include serving as director of the University of Oklahoma Graduate Program, Tulsa campus; director of the Harris School of Nursing, TCU; and dean of the Harris College, TCU. During her administrative career, she has focused on creating new educational pathways and opportunities in higher education for nurses and health professionals.

Sister Rosemary Donley, PhD, APRN, BC, FAAN

Sister Rosemary Donley, a Sister of Charity of Seton Hill, is a professor of nursing and the Jacques Laval Chair for Justice for Vulnerable Populations at Duquesne University School of Nursing. She received a diploma from the Pittsburgh Hospital School of Nursing and holds a bachelor of science in nursing (summa cum laude) from St. Louis University and a master of nursing education and a PhD from the University of Pittsburgh. She is a certified adult nurse practitioner with clinical and research interests directed to improving the lives of vulnerable people.

Prior to coming to Duquesne in 2009, Sr. Rosemary was dean of nursing, executive vice president of the university, and director of graduate programs in community/public health nursing at The Catholic University of America (CUA).

Sr. Rosemary has served as president of the National League for Nursing and Sigma Theta Tau International Honor Society of Nursing. She was a Robert Wood Johnson Health Policy Fellow and is a past senior editor of *Image: The Journal of Nursing Scholarship*. She is a member of the Department of Veterans Affairs' Special Medical Advisory Group and of the Board of Directors of the Commission on Graduates of Foreign Nurse Schools (CGFNS). She is a member of the Institute of Medicine and the American Academy of Nursing. A recipient of seven honorary degrees, she has received the Nell J. Watts Lifetime Achievement in Nursing Award and the Elizabeth Seton Medal.

David Anthony (Tony) Forrester, PhD, RN, ANEF

Tony Forrester is professor and senior associate dean for Academic Affairs and Administration in the School of Nursing at Rutgers University (formerly the University of Medicine and Dentistry of New Jersey [UMDNJ]) and is clinical professor in the Department of Environmental Medicine at Rutgers' Robert Wood Johnson Medical School (RWJMS). He is also professor in residence and an interdisciplinary health research consultant at Morristown Medical Center.

Forrester graduated from the University of Texas System School of Nursing (1975; Fort Worth) with a bachelor of science in nursing, from the University of Texas at Arlington with a master of science in nursing (1979; Arlington), and from New York University with a PhD in research and theory development in nursing (1984; New York). Forrester is a widely known scholar, serves as a peer reviewer for a number of professional/scholarly nursing journals, and has published extensively on a wide range of topics, including HIV/AIDS; critical care family needs; aggressiveness of nursing care at the end of life; gender-related health, including minority men's and women's health; falls risk assessment and prevention in the acute care setting; physical restraints management; and nursing history. He is a fellow in the National League for Nursing's Academy of Nursing Education. He is an active member of a number of professional and scholarly associations, including the American Nurses Association, New Jersey State Nurses Association, and Sigma Theta Tau International (STTI). Forrester is currently serving as the leader for eight international expert faculty members in the STTI Nurse Faculty Leadership Academy (NFLA).

Esther C. Gallegos, PhD

Dr. Esther Gallegos has been a faculty member of the College of Nursing, Universidad Autónoma de Nuevo León, in Monterrey, Nueva León, México, since 1969 and has taught in undergraduate and graduate nursing programs. At the graduate level, she led the building of the curriculum for the master and doctoral programs. Both programs have been pioneers in nursing education in Mexico. At the Universidad Autónoma de Nuevo León, Gallegos has held administrative and academic positions as the dean of the College of Nursing and membership in the government council of the university.

Gallegos has also developed international work in Latin America through diverse academic and research projects as well as serving as a keynote speaker. Her research area is self-care in chronic diseases, including risk factors prevention.

In 1998, Gallegos, nursing emerita, received the national award Isabel Cendala y Gómez from the Health Secretariat Council of Mexico. She is an elected fellow of the American Academy of Nursing and a member of the National System of Researchers in Mexico.

Jennifer Gray, PhD, RN

Jennifer Gray is interim dean of the University of Texas at Arlington College of Nursing and remains associate dean for the MSN Administration, Education, and PhD programs. On UTA's faculty since 1989, she has taught in all programs at the college and has won several teaching awards. Gray holds a BSN from the University of Central Oklahoma, an MSN from the University of Texas at Arlington, and a PhD with a focus on theory development and research from Texas Woman's University, Denton. Gray has conducted studies on HIV/AIDS medication adherence, knowledge of perinatal HIV care, and quality of work life of nurses in Uganda. As the George W. and Hazel M. Jay Professor, she has worked with a team of nurses in Uganda developing research capacity

Manuel Moreno, PhD

Dr. Manuel Moreno graduated with a degree in nursing in 1983 from the École Le Bon Secours (Geneva, Switzerland). In 2000, he obtained the degree of Social and Cultural Anthropology at the University of San Antonio (Spain), and in 2006 he completed his PhD at the same university with research about the relationship between nursing professionals and immigrant patients. He began his career as a teacher in 1998 at the Universidad Europea de Madrid, teaching a variety of subjects. Between

2007 and 2012, he was head of the Nursing Department at the university. He is a reviewer for several publications and scientific societies in the area of nursing and anthropology. He has written more than 25 papers in scientific journals and is author of a book titled *El Cuidado de Otro*.

He is currently the titular professor at Universidad Europea de Madrid in Madrid, Spain. He is an honorary member of the Delta Theta Chapter of Sigma Theta Tau International.

Karen H. Morin, DSN, RN, ANEF, FAAN

Dr. Karen Morin is a professor of nursing at the University of Wisconsin–Milwaukee, where she serves as director of the PhD program. Over the course of the last 30 years, Morin has held teaching positions at the University of Alabama at Birmingham, Thomas Jefferson University, Widener University, Pennsylvania State University, and Western Michigan University.

Not only has Morin published more than 100 journal articles, chapters, and abstracts, she also has been recognized for her teaching abilities. She received the Excellence in Teaching Award from the National League for Nursing in 2003 and the Excellence in Nursing Education Award from the Association of Women's Health, Obstetric, and Neonatal Nurses in 1999. She has given numerous presentations addressing the need for practice based on evidence, the need for leadership succession planning, and the influence of mentorship on the profession. She has been actively involved in several Sigma Theta Tau International (STTI) leadership programs, such as Board Leadership, and is a founding faculty member of the Sigma Theta Tau International and Johnson & Johnson Maternal-Child Health Nurse Leadership Academy.

She has held leadership positions in STTI since her induction, having served as chapter president for two chapters as well as founding president of another chapter. She has also served on numerous international committees. As president of STTI, she was instrumental in procuring nongovernmental organization (NGO) associative status for the organization, in supporting the organization's momentum in becoming truly global, and for increasing the opportunity for members' voices outside North America to be heard.

Morin holds a bachelor's degree from the University of Ottawa, Ottawa, Ontario, Canada; a master of science in nursing from the University of Central Arkansas; and a doctorate of science in nursing (DNS) from the University of Alabama at Birmingham. She is a fellow in the Academy of Nurse Educators (ANEF) and the American Academy of Nursing (FAAN).

Roberta K. Olson, PhD, RN

Dr. Roberta K. Olson holds a bachelor of science in nursing from South Dakota State University; a master of science in nursing from Washington University, St. Louis; and a PhD in organization and administration of higher education from Saint Louis University.

Since 1994, Olson has served as the dean of nursing at South Dakota State University in Brookings. She has been successful in working with the college development officer to bring in significant scholarship and program support for the College of Nursing.

Olson is the author of several publications in the areas of nursing education, nursing of children, and mentoring in nursing. She coauthored *The Mentor Connection in Nursing* with Dr. Connie Vance, which was published in 1998 by Springer Publishing.

Franklin A. Shaffer, EdD, RN, FAAN

Dr. Franklin A. Shaffer is the chief executive officer of Commission on Graduates of Foreign Nursing Schools International (CGFNS), the world's largest credentials evaluation organization for nursing. CGFNS is an immigration neutral, nonprofit organization founded in 1977 and based in Philadelphia, Pennsylvania. CGFNS is internationally recognized as the leading authority on education, registration, and licensure of nurses worldwide.

He earned his doctorate in education at Teacher's College, Columbia University. Shaffer was awarded an honorary doctorate of science at Cedar Crest College. He has authored and edited six books as well as numerous chapters in other works and serves on the editorial boards of several leading professional journals. He has more than 40 years of progressive and varied nursing experience, including administration, education, clinical, and research. He was appointed to the Joint Commission's Nursing Advisory Council, where he made the business case for the Joint Commission to establish the health care staffing industry certification program.

Shaffer is the past president of the Friends of the National Institute for Nursing Research. Shaffer is a member of the American Organization of Nurse Executive's (AONE) editorial board for the journal *Nurse Leader* as well as the editorial board of *Nursing Administration Quarterly* and American Nurses Association's (ANA) *American Nurse Today*. He is a frequent speaker at domestic conferences/conventions. He provided consultation services and lectured in the Netherlands, the United Kingdom, Germany, Brazil, Japan, and Korea. Shaffer served on the Happtique's Blue Ribbon Panel to develop a certification program for mobile health applications.

Shaffer is a fellow of the American Academy of Nursing and a recipient of the most distinguished R. Louise McManus Medal from Columbia University for his contributions to the profession.

Patricia E. Thompson, EdD, RN, FAAN

Dr. Patricia E. Thompson is CEO of Sigma Theta Tau International. She began her clinical career as a pediatric staff nurse. The majority of her career has been academically based in faculty and administrator roles, and she has been an investigator of numerous grant-funded programs. Thompson has published and presented on leadership, scholarship, maternal-child issues, and nursing education. She has also served on professional and community boards.

Connie Vance, EdD, RN, FAAN

Dr. Connie Vance is professor and former dean at the College of New Rochelle School of Nursing, New Rochelle, New York. Vance is a fellow of the American Academy of Nursing, fellow of the New York Academy of Medicine, member of the Nursing Hall of Fame at Columbia University, and honorary member of the American Association of Colleges of Nursing. Her research and writing are in the areas of mentorship, leadership development, global affairs, and public policy.

Vance serves on several professional and editorial boards, including *Nursing Spectrum* of NY/NJ, *Nursing Economics*, and *Journal of Dokuz Eylul University School of Nursing*, Izmir, Turkey. She is cofounder of the Global Society for Nursing and Health, trustee of Hope for a Healthier Humanity, and an honorary member of the Russian Association of Educators of Nursing and Pharmaceutical Colleges.

Her publications include *Fast Facts for Career Success in Nursing: Making the Most of Mentoring* (2011) and *The Mentor Connection in Nursing* (1998).

She is a member of the International Mentoring Association, Global Task Force of the American Academy of Nursing, and Leadership Roundtable at the New York Academy of Medicine. Vance serves as a consultant to professional nursing associations, educational programs, and hospital nursing departments throughout the United States and internationally.

Table of Contents

Foreword

Patricia E. Thompson, EdD, RN, FAAN

When I was asked to write a foreword to *Mentoring Today's Nurses: A Global Perspective for Success*, I was delighted for two reasons: the topic—mentoring—and Mary Lou Bond, PhD, RN, CNE, ANEF, FAAN. Mentoring played a key role in my professional development, as it did for most of my nurse colleagues. As a student, I had a faculty mentor who encouraged me to get my master's degree and consider teaching. Later, as a novice faculty member in my first teaching position, Dr. Bond was my mentor. With her guidance, I, too, became an effective teacher and mentor. Mary Lou and I have maintained a personal and professional relationship for more than 35 years.

I was fortunate to have other mentors, too. In fact, I would not be the chief executive officer of the Honor Society of Nursing, Sigma Theta Tau International (STTI) had it not been for the nurturing and prodding of many mentors throughout my career. Because of my experience, I recognize how important it is to the future of our profession that we mentor others, especially students and new graduates. Therefore, I am committed to mentoring these groups, as well as others, every time I have an opportunity to do so. As I stated in a column that I wrote for *Reflections on Nursing Leadership*, STTI's online magazine:

> As mentors, we need to support students and newly graduated nurses so they will become confident leaders, whether at the point of care or in roles that influence the point of care—at the bedside, in the community, at the board table, and around the world. This process takes time, because many new nurses don't consider themselves leaders and, without help from a mentor, don't recognize their potential.

When it comes to mentoring globally, we encounter differences in cultures and traditions, and it may be more difficult for a mentor from one country or geographic region to effectively assist a mentee from another part of the world. This book addresses those gaps by showing you how to build bridges of effective communication.

But you don't have to travel outside your native country to recognize the value of the content and practical tips presented in this book.

With current technology and travel availability, we are truly a global community. Most countries have multicultural populations, and the rich diversity of a nation's people is reflected in its educational institutions, health care workforce, and patient base. Mentors need to be aware of and understand the cultural values and traditions of their mentees. For example, gender roles and power-base differences within a society create a cultural milieu that has significant implications for mentor-mentee relationships.

The authors of *Mentoring Today's Nurses: A Global Perspective for Success* will help you navigate as seamlessly as possible from culture to culture. Each one of them is an expert educator and mentor with broad global experience, and they combine in-depth content with personal examples to engage the reader. In addition, the Global Mentoring Process Model provides a framework for understanding the culture and traditions of mentoring.

We all have a responsibility to mentor the future leaders of our profession, who come from a variety of cultural backgrounds. Nurse educators working with students, at all levels, and clinical managers working with new graduates will benefit greatly from the wealth of information found in this book.

Foreword

Karen H. Morin, DSN, RN, ANEF, FAAN

The process of mentoring and the persons involved in the process (mentor and mentee) have received considerable attention in the literature for more than 50 years. Even after so many years, academic interest in mentoring remains high: a quick search of Medline using the key word "mentoring" yielded 8,784 hits; using the key words "mentoring in nursing" yielded 2,925 hits. In nursing, mentoring has been examined in terms of RN-to-FNP transition (Poronsky, 2012), faculty development (Gwyn, 2011; Heinrich & Oberleitner, 2012; Nick et al., 2012; Salma, Hegadoren, & Ogilvie, 2012; Slimmer, 2012), undergraduate student transition (Kostovich & Thurn, 2013; Omer, Suliman, Thomas, & Joseph, 2013), international research collaboration (Anderson, Friedemann, Büscher, Sansoni, & Hodnicki, 2012), and recruitment of minority students (Rearden, 2012). Mentors are being used to support nurses whose practices have been questioned (Sprinks, 2012) and to help infuse evidence-based practice into health care systems (Jeffers, Robinson, Luxner, & Redding, 2008). The role mentors can play has been discussed in relation to translational scientist development (Pfund et al., 2013) as well as in the development of biostatisticians (Odueyunhbo & Thabane, 2012).

This text places the topic of mentoring within a global context and within a specific model of mentoring, the Global Mentoring Process Model, which is discussed in Chapter 1. The authors have adapted a model to better reflect their perspective of mentoring and the impact that mentoring has on the discipline. Of note is the emphasis placed on the contribution nursing science offers to mentoring. Personal narratives make the concept of mentoring more meaningful within the context of the model.

The authors have devoted considerable discussion to how mentoring can be undertaken within educational institutions, including challenges for students and faculty. Of critical importance is the discussion about how mentoring is perceived and made operational in select countries outside the United States. In Chapter 7, Jennifer Gray, Manuel Moreno, and Esther C. Gallegos share that mentoring takes different forms, depending on the country in which it is being implemented, and offer valuable advice to readers along with some relevant examples. This information becomes critical when undertaking mentoring relationships with colleagues, students, practitioners, or scientists from countries other than one's own.

This book promises to challenge the reader to think in new and different ways about the opportunities that mentoring can offer. Certainly, we are up to the challenge!

References

Anderson, K. H., Friedemann, M. L., Büscher, A., Sansoni, J., & Hodnicki, D. (2012). Immersion research education: Students as catalysts in international collaboration research. *Nursing Review, 59*, 502–510.

Gwyn, P. G. (2011). The quality of mentoring relationships' impact on the occupational commitment of nursing faculty. *Journal of Professional Nursing, 27*, 292–298. doi:10.1016/j. profnurs.2011.03.008

Heinrich, K. T., & Oberleitner, M. G. (2012). How a faculty group's peer mentoring of each other's scholarship can enhance retention and recruitment. *Journal of Professional Nursing, 28*, 5–12. doi:10.1016/j.profnurs.2011.06.002

Jeffers, B., Robinson, S., Luxner, K., & Redding, D. (2008). Nursing faculty mentors as facilitators for evidence-based nursing practice. *Journal for Nurses in Staff Development, 24*(5), E8–E12.

Kostovich, C. T., & Thurn, K. E. (2013). Group mentoring: A story of transition for undergraduate baccalaureate nursing students. *Nurse Education Today, 33*(4), 314–418. doi:org/10.1016/j. nedt.2012.12.016

Nick, J. M., Delahoyde, T. M., Del Prato, D., Mitchell, C., Ortiz, J., Ottley, C., . . . Siktberg, L. (2012). Best practices in academic mentoring: A model of excellence. *Nursing Research and Practice,* article ID 937906, 2012, 1–9. doi:10.2255/2012/937906

Odueyungbo, A., & Thabane, L. (2012). Mentoring in biostatistics: Some suggestions for reform. *Journal of Multidisciplinary Healthcare, 5*, 265–272.

Omer, T. Y., Suliman, W. A., Thomas, L., & Joseph, J. (2013). Perception of nursing students to two models of preceptorship in clinical training. *Nurse Education in Practice*, 1–6. http://dx.doi.org/10.1016/j,nepr.2013.02.003

Pfund, C., House, S., Spencer, K., Asquith, P., Carney, P., Masters, K. S., . . . Fleming, M. (2013). A research mentor training curriculum for clinical and translational researchers. *Clinical and Translational Science, 6*, 25–33. doi:10.1111/cts.12009

Poronsky, C. B. (2012). A literature review of mentoring for RN-to-FNP transition. *Journal of Nursing Education, 51*, 623–631. doi:10.3928/01484834-20120914-03

Rearden, A. K. (2012). Recruitment and retention of Alaska natives into nursing: Elements enabling educational success. *Journal of Cultural Diversity, 19*, 72–78.

Salma, J., Hegadoren, K. M., & Ogilvie, L. (2012). Career advancement and educational opportunities: Experiences and perceptions of internationally educated nurses. *Nursing Leadership, 25*(3), 56–67.

Slimmer, L. (2012). A teaching mentorship program to facilitate excellence in teaching and learning. *Journal of Professional Nursing, 28*, 182–185. Doi:10.1016/j.profnurs.2011.11.006

Sprinks, J. (2012). RCN will offer mentor support to nurses facing misconduct charges. *Nursing Standard, 27*(5), 5.

Foreword

Connie Vance, EdD, RN, FAAN

The broad sweep of mentorship in the nursing profession presented in this practical and informative book is evidence that nurses are actively involved in mentor relationships at every level, specialty, and locale. Whether through the academic experience, the workplace, or professional associations, nurses around the world have begun to understand that mentor connections are essential to professional success—as individuals and as a profession. Nurses have come a long way in their knowledge of mentoring since the mid 1970's, when the word *mentor* was absent from the profession's vocabulary. Our voices about mentoring were silent, albeit we engaged in preceptoring and role modeling for professional development.

The first formal investigation of mentoring in nursing was conducted with contemporary leaders, known as "nurse influentials" (Vance, 1977), and there were some surprises. In spite of the scarcity of formal mentoring in the profession, these nursing leaders asserted that they had indeed received substantial mentoring assistance from various sources throughout their productive careers. Further, as they were successful in their leadership journey, they served as mentors to the next generation of nurses. These successful leaders lived, learned, and worked in the presence of strong, abiding mentor relationships that served as a source of power and influence for them and their work. Their protégés, in turn, have mentored generations of nurses in expanding spheres of achievement and influenced nursing and health care around the world. Thus, one of the principles of mentoring was demonstrated in this study, i.e., that those who are mentored will mentor others, in a generational pattern, thus expanding future knowledge, leadership, and change. Mentoring is always about the future and dreams for a better future.

In our contemporary world, every nurse is called to lead. We are challenged to be transformative leaders who "lead change and advance health" (Institute of Medicine, 2010, p. S–3). Our mentor connections will be a key factor in developing a broad talent pool of transformative leaders who can deliver innovative, humanistic care to people. Our mentor connections will allow us to expand our spheres of influence in all sectors of society, and to be policy activists and change makers. Mentoring networks will strengthen our endeavors to redesign and advance cutting edge health care approaches in our country and around the world. We simply cannot be influential transformative leaders unless we intentionally and deliberately mentor each other at every stage of our challenging work. This means that every student and every nurse must see themselves as both mentors and protégés. Each student and each professional nurse has something valuable to offer his or her peers and colleagues behind and ahead of them. Likewise, each of us needs mentoring guidance that will inspire us to make important contributions in society. This is reciprocal mutuality in which all who enter the mentor relationship will receive the enormous benefits of networking and support. This mutuality ultimately will create an ever-expanding source of knowledge, motivation, and advocacy for each other, for the profession, and ultimately for the people we serve.

Mentor connections are developmental and empowering relationships that entail intentional mutual sharing, learning, and growth (Vance & Olson, 1998). We create broad networks of multiple and diverse mentoring opportunities and mentor relationships throughout the entire trajectory of our careers. I call this "power mentoring." This concept is amply demonstrated in this important book. The editors and authors provide a broad array of anecdotal and empirical data, evidence-based mentoring, best practices, models, and guidelines for expanding our mentor connections. They bring a "local" and "cosmopolitan" worldview to the nursing profession and to nurses' activities as mentors and protégés. I applaud this book and its contributors for the wisdom and guidance they present in helping us become better mentor-leaders—and transformative visionaries who inspire, guide, and advocate for each other and our work. Nurses are natural mentors. They embody compassion and generosity. These qualities can be applied to mentoring each other for the realization of our enormous potential. Nursing's powerhouse of talent must be unleashed to "lead change and advance health."

This book amply demonstrates how broadly and deeply nurses can mentor each other. We can do it through our daily contacts; we can mentor through formal planned programs that match mentors and protégés in a guided process. Nurses can mentor each other in expert-to-novice or peer-to-peer models. We can engage in collective mentoring (particularly in academe, research programs, and nursing associations) and e-mentoring (particularly in global work). We can develop long-term mentoring relationships that may last a lifetime or in short-term, "one-minute" mentoring encounters. Nurses can introduce novices to the profession through intentional informal and formal mentoring. Nurses can activate succession planning by identifying talent and mentoring that talent for the next generation of professional innovation. Mentor-leaders can create a culture of mentorship in schools, the workplace, and professional associations. Nurses must seek mentors in every career stage to guide them as they enter a new specialty, a new challenge, or a new turn in their career journey. The possibilities are endless and exciting. This book challenges each of us to activate mentoring as a local and global endeavor and provides important guidance for our success as transformative mentor–leaders.

References

Institute of Medicine. (2010). *The future of nursing: Leading change, advancing health*. Washington, DC: 2010.

Vance, C. (1977). *A group profile of contemporary influentials in American nursing* (doctoral dissertation). Retrieved from ProQuest, University Microforms International Dissertations Publishing. (7804472).

Vance, C. & Olson, R. K. (Eds.). (1998). *The mentor connection in nursing*. New York, NY: Springer.

Foreword

Franklin A. Shaffer EdD, RN, FAAN

Whether formal or informal, mentoring demands that one person reach out to another in a sincere attempt to help him or her advance in a chosen career. This desire to help must not be condescending but offered freely from a heart full of gratitude to all those who have helped the mentor in the past—for, as any honest person readily admits, no one succeeds without help. When reaching out to someone of another culture, one assumes a number of responsibilities; the first is to make an effort to appreciate the culture, for it provides a blueprint to understanding the internationally educated nurse's (IEN) thoughts, behaviors, and choices. However, not every person in a culture ascribes to all or even part of its tenets; and even if both mentor and mentee are from the same culture, their belief systems may differ greatly. What we call "cultural competence" is far more complex than learning cultural stereotypes: It also requires respect for the mentee's individuality, and demands openness to learning and the patience to work through the inevitable gaffes.

Many IENs will not speak up initially, so paying close attention to their body language is essential. A "language barrier" includes conversational styles and customs as well as idioms, eye contact, dialects, pacing, and the fear of being thought ignorant. Explaining slang, irony, and humor helps mentees understand the meaning and context of the spoken word, and addressing these matters early greatly improves the mentee's experience. Speaking a second language, especially one learned as an adult, is difficult. By comparison, reading the language tends to be easier, so always provide critical information in writing.

According to Benner (1984), discovering nurses' assumptions, expectations, and skill sets and uncovering unexpected differences in practical knowledge are essential aspects of mentoring. Few tasks are as difficult as changing the way you have learned to practice. As Susan Baxley, Kristina Ibitayo, and Mary Lou Bond point out in Chapter 1, the mentee could be a U.S. nurse who is working in another culture: "As the only American nurse in the hospital, I depended heavily on support from the nurses, the nurse aides, and the hospital physician to help me learn what to do and what not to do" (p. 10). Other significant challenges include gender relationships, physical assessment skills, pharmacology (the names of common drugs differ from country to country), and the role of the nurse in a practice setting. Time-management practices and the ability to properly set priorities also must be explored and explained (Williams, 1992).

Helping mentees develop professional networks may be the best contribution that mentors can make. Mentors should start by ensuring that mentees make contact with others in their own cultures and have identified a church, a synagogue, or a mosque near where they live to significantly reduce stress levels and increase the ability to acclimate more quickly. However, mentees still need to learn new cultures and new systems. Mentors must find relevant people and introduce their mentees to them. Building a network is so important that CGFNS International is moving from being a one-time "entry service" to a lifelong resource for migrating professionals. We started an Educational Institute to help CGFNS International become a career center for immigrant nurses, providing upward mobility through online remediation, education, career coaches, and mentors. This will be done through leveraging the intellectual capital of CGFNS staff, and through the development of a collaborative network between CGFNS University and leading universities in the United States.

There is a small but growing body of literature on the subject of mentoring IENs, not least of which is the International Center on Migration's book on individual best practices for helping IENs adapt to their new culture: *The Official Guide for Foreign-Educated Nurses: What You Need to Know About Nursing and Health Care in the United States* (Springer Publishing Company, 2009). CGFNS has sponsored research on IENs' profiles ("Characteristics of International Practical Nurses Graduates in the Unites States Workforce, 2003–2004" [Commission on Graduates of Foreign Nursing Schools, 2005]), which some mentors might find very useful. Moreover, the International Centre on Nurse Migration publishes a newsletter called *ICNM News* that contains pertinent information, up-to-date news, and useful resources and links.

The authors in this book explore these issues and many more, and they offer sound advice based on their personal and professional experiences. In its own way, this book "mentors" the mentors who will be guiding the next generation.

References

Benner, P. (1984). *From novice to expert: Excellence and power in clinical nursing practice.* Menlo Park, CA: Addison-Wesley.

Williams, J. (1992). Orienting foreign nurse graduates through preceptors. *Journal of Nursing Staff Development, 8*(3), 155–158.

Introduction

There is no greater accomplishment for mentors than
when people they develop pass them by!

–John C. Maxwell

The focus of this book is mentoring within educational and health care settings, where nursing students and professional nurses must learn how to assess and negotiate multiple systems. Entering a new system, whether it is an educational environment or a health care environment, is conceptualized as a new culture. This book discusses various perspectives of mentoring, and, as the individual reader reflects upon the provided TIPS (thoughts, ideas, possible strategies), it presents strategies unique to each person regarding how to maximize the mentoring experience within a specific mentor structure.

In this book, we have provided practical advice for how to mentor students at all levels within the educational system as well as new and seasoned nurses within health care systems as they assume new roles. Mentees/protégés will learn how to request and apply guidance from their mentors. Students will also receive advice on seeking out mentors and resolving issues when the relationships are not meeting their needs. As the environments in which we find ourselves become increasingly global, students and nurses in the United States and those coming to the United States have a variety of expectations and fears coupled with cultural, gender, and religious considerations that affect how they will function in a new society.

Although mentoring has been defined in many ways, and means different things to different people, most disciplines/professions have mentoring activities to assist those who are new in their roles. The process of mentoring individuals from within and from without the United States, conceptualized as *global mentoring*, results from having a reciprocal, mutually beneficial relationship between a mentor and a protégé that challenges and is based on trust, communication, respect, and cultural influences.

The goal of this book is to inform nurses about mentoring practices for nursing students in a variety of academic programs, new graduates, and seasoned nurses who move from one role to another in today's complex health care systems. Helpful hints for protégés looking for and working with mentors are also offered. Additionally, this book provides practical information for how to provide support for international students and professional nurses who choose to practice in the United States. If international students and nurses are to be successful and contribute to nursing practice and science, it is important to understand what is expected in the way of support and guidance from professionals with whom they will associate. Although the mentor/protégé relationship may vary from country to country, it also reflects commonalities, such as the concepts within the Global Mentoring Process Model.

Because mentoring has been identified as critical to professional success in many disciplines, this book informs a variety of nurses who struggle to support students and colleagues along the continuum of nursing education and as they enter practice. It provides practical information to those who struggle to understand the patterns and expectations of students at all levels, as well as new and seasoned professional nurses within a global society as they move from one location to another and from one role to similar or dissimilar ones.

Faculty and students in all schools of nursing and health professions in the United States, Canada, England, and other countries where English is spoken and clinicians and administrators in hospitals throughout these same countries will benefit from this book. The American Hospital Association and Magnet hospitals, in particular, will benefit from the content of the book as they work to mentor new nurses and health care workers.

Chapter 1 describes the Global Mentoring Process Model—a two-way process that requires the essential components of mutual benefit, respect, trust, cultural influences, communication, and challenge—and its contribution to nursing science. The volume editors reflect on their experiences of being mentored.

Chapter 2 provides an overview of systems, from the mechanistic worldview and general systems theory to the more current worldview of complexity theory, which focuses on complex adaptive systems. Suggestions for negotiating various systems are offered.

Chapter 3 presents selected challenges of the educational system to students, from a faculty perspective. Examples of challenges for BSN, RN-to-BSN, MSN, PhD, and DNP students are discussed.

Chapter 4 discusses the challenges of the educational system to faculty. Challenges for faculty to address the needs of students at various levels of studies are compared and contrasted. The chapter also provides suggestions for navigating educational systems.

Chapter 5 provides a detailed description of the challenges inherent in mentoring faculty at all levels, along with tips for mentorship. Selected resources available to assist those who mentor faculty colleagues are summarized.

Chapter 6 offers insights into the need for mentors within today's health care systems for new graduates, seasoned professionals who move into new roles, and international nurses entering the U.S. health care system. English as a second language and the nuances of communication, as well as differing nursing cultures within their systems, are explored.

Chapter 7 presents what nurse faculty from selected countries report on global mentoring traditions, which include both differences and commonalities from around the world. The ways in which mentoring is experienced and implemented, mentor and mentee roles, and the ways that cultural values influence a mentoring relationship are explored.

Chapter 8 shares the reflections of two former presidents of Sigma Theta Tau International based on their personal and professional experiences.

The epilogue summarizes various authors' personal reflections to confirm the key concepts within the Global Mentoring Process Model and explore the ways nurses have become a major force in influencing the science of nursing.

Appendix A offers a list of selected resources and available websites, including examples from the United States, Spanish-language websites, and a variety of countries within different Sigma Theta Tau International regions throughout the world.

It is our hope that as we have been challenged and mentored, readers will be challenged to reflect on their own experiences and how they in turn can mentor the next generation of nurses. This shared responsibility will allow us to become transformative leaders in an increasingly global society.

The mentoring bracelet (Figure i.1), worn every day by Bond, is a constant reminder of the multiple mentors in her life. Without individuals from various institutions nationally and globally, she would not have been able to negotiate the complex systems she found while studying, working, and moving from one state and country to another. Other individuals may have specific mementos that remind of them of their mentoring experiences. Additionally, nursing organizations— such as the Southern Nursing Research Society, for instance— have pins that members may provide as gifts to their mentors in appreciation for their assistance.

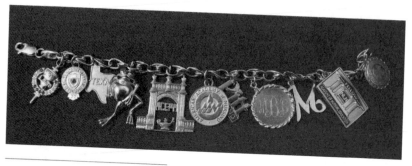

FIGURE i.1

Mary Lou Bond's Mentoring Bracelet

From left to right are symbols of organizations/individuals who served as mentors to Mary Lou: leaders of Sigma Theta Tau International, faculty colleagues from the University of Texas at Arlington, nurse and faculty colleagues from throughout Texas, faculty/mentors from Puerto Rico, nurse colleagues from Mexico, mentors in the American Academy of Nursing, faculty/mentors from the University of Pittsburgh, faculty/

mentors from Texas Christian University, dissertation chair, mentors/colleagues from the Academy of Nurse Educators, and mentors from Bethel Deaconess Hospital.

And a second author shares her reflections on mentoring.

Reflections on Mentoring
By Kristina S. Ibitayo, PhD, RN

My mentor, her mentor, our mentors,
Individualized experiences,
Contextual differences.

Reflections on mentoring
Affirm memorable connections,
Signal change, growth, and
Outcomes of choices made.

Simple, yet profound,
The effect of mentors,
On protégés' myriad journeys.
Time tells the story.

Chapter 1
Global Mentoring: Guiding Hands

Susan M. Baxley, Kristina S. Ibitayo, and Mary Lou Bond

Mentoring means different things to each of us. Some may not even realize that mentoring has occurred, whereas others clearly recall the distinct impact mentoring relationships have made in their lives. Some protégés go through the whole mentoring process feeling as if they are in the care of guiding hands. Just as each person has a distinct life journey, personal experiences with mentoring also vary. There is the stage of mentoring where we are passive recipients, the stage where we seek guidance but offer little to the mentor, and the stage where mentors and protégés have give-and-take relationships in which both participants receive what they want and need from the relationship (Grossman, 2007). The mentoring process is cyclical, as each individual progresses through the stages of mentoring; a protégé may simultaneously be another person's mentor and participate in a mentoring network (Grossman, 2013). Not all mentoring relationships endure or remain unchanged. If the mentoring relationship no longer is working or has reached fulfillment for either protégé or mentor, it is time to move on to other relationships.

This chapter presents a conceptual framework of the Global Mentoring Process Model based upon our personal reflections and adaption of Zey's (1991) Mutual Benefits Model. The context of "global" is in a universal mentoring process that encompasses nurses across varied cultures from within and outside the United States (U.S.). The term "global" is based in the reality of today's contemporary world and the necessity of globalization to maintain a competitive edge in today's marketplace. Globalization is "the shift toward a more integrated and interdependent world economy" (Hill, 2013, p. 6). The globalization trend in health care is present today in some activities and procedures, such as radiology interpretation and in medical tourists' undergoing surgical procedures outside the United States (Hill, 2013). Due to the globalization process and advances in telecommunication technology and transportation, the challenges associated with such barriers as distance and differences in time zones and language have decreased (Hill, 2013). In the global context of mentoring, nursing colleagues from around the world interact with nurses from other countries in the workplace and at nursing conferences, benefiting from the expansion of nursing knowledge as they learn from one another.

Zey's Mutual Benefits Model is a business mentoring model focusing on the mentor and protégé relationship and positive organizational results. We have used Zey's conceptual structure of the mentor and protégé being a mutually beneficial relationship. In Zey's model, the mentoring relationship only benefits the organization, whereas in our model, the mentor-protégé relationship contributes to the science of nursing through the mentoring structures. The science of nursing in turn provides the mentoring dyads with knowledge, culture, professional networks, and resources to assist the protégés and mentors in personal and professional development. Zey's concepts of knowledge, personal support, prestige, and protection are included in our model, and support for these concepts is found in current nursing literature (Anibas, Brenner, & Zorn, 2009; Dunham-Taylor, Lynn, Moore, McDaniel, & Walker, 2008; Elcigil & Sari, 2008; Erdem & Aytemur, 2008; Huybrecht, Loeckx, Quaeyhaegens, Tobel, & Mistiaen, 2011; Jakubik, 2008; McGuire & Reger, 2003; Nies & Troutman-Jordan, 2012).

As the mentoring relationship develops, a structure is chosen and followed by both participants; however, the structure may change as the relationship blossoms or wanes. The process of global mentoring (Figure 1.1) occurs as a result of having a reciprocal, mutually beneficial relationship between a mentor and a protégé that challenges and is based on trust, communication, respect, and cultural influences (Jakubik, 2008; Zey, 1991). This process benefits the science of nursing (Jakubik, Eliades, Gavriloff, & Weese, 2011; Nies & Troutman-Jordan, 2012) by promoting the key factors that occur within the context of the mentor-protégé relationship—namely, knowledge, personal/emotional support, advancement, expertise, protection, loyalty, prestige, and role models (Anibas et al., 2009; Dunham-Taylor et al., 2008; Elcigil & Sari, 2008; Erdem & Aytemur, 2008; Huybrecht et al., 2011; McGuire & Reger, 2003; Nies & Troutman-Jordan, 2012). The process can have varied mentoring structures, such as formal, informal (Grossman, 2013), co-mentoring/peer (Heinrich & Oberleitner, 2012; McGuire & Reger, 2003), e-mentoring (Klein, 2003), coaching (Gibson & Heartfield, 2005), and/or cascade mentoring (Walker, Golde, Jones, Bueschel, & Hutchings, 2008). These different types of structures can occur within academic and health care systems.

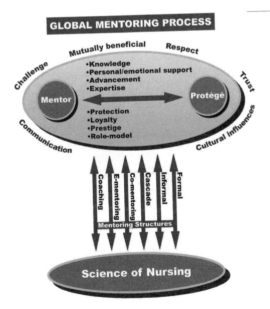

FIGURE 1.1

Global Mentoring Process Model. Baxley & Ibitayo (2012). Adapted from Zey's (1991) Mutual Benefits Model. From unpublished model, by S. Baxley and K. Ibitayo, 2012. Copyright 2012 by copyright holders. Reprinted with permission.

The mentoring relationship is a two-way process that requires the essential components of mutual benefits, respect, trust, cultural influences, communication, and challenges. Nursing scholars have different definitions of nursing (Barrett, 2002; Fawcett, 2012), so there is no one definition of nursing science. For this model, we use the definition of nursing science provided by the American Academy of Nursing's Expert Panel on Nursing Theory–Guided Practice to provide a foundation for our thinking on how the science of nursing influences the Global Mentoring Process Model within nursing:

Nursing science is the substantive discipline-specific knowledge that focuses on the human-universe-health process articulated in the nursing frameworks and theories. The discipline-specific knowledge reflects the philosophical perspectives embedded in the ontological, epistemological, and methodological processes that frame nursing's ethical approach to the human-universe-health process (Parse et al., 2000, p. 177).

Our conceptual framework views the science of nursing as supporting and providing context for each dyad with the knowledge, culture, professional network, and resources necessary for the mentor and protégé to experience professional and personal growth (Holmes, Hodgson, Simari, & Nishimura, 2010; Jakubik, 2008; Zey, 1991). Some protégés who are experts in their fields of nursing may not require the same level or type of mentoring structure as a novice nurse. The six mentoring structures (formal, informal, cascade, co-mentoring, e-mentoring, and coaching) provide the mechanism to influence and support the science of nursing and the mentor-protégé dyad.

The six structural mentoring definitions are as follows:

- Formal mentoring "occurs when an institution implements a formally recognized mentoring scheme" (Gibson & Heartfield, 2005, p. 52).

- Informal mentoring is "when one person takes an interest in the well-being and advancement of another" (Gibson & Heartfield, 2005, p. 51).

- Co-mentoring is noncompetitive (Grossman, 2013), offers a "safe space to take intellectual and emotional risks," and is role affirming and nurturing (McGuire & Reger, 2003, p. 65). The term *co-mentor* is synonymous with peers and buddies (Grossman, 2013).

- Coaching is the "process of equipping people with the tools, knowledge, and opportunities they need to develop themselves and become more effective" (Peterson & Hicks, 1996, p. 41).

- E-mentoring provides online resources and the ability to connect and form a virtual community (Klein, 2003) with people of similar interests.

- Cascade mentoring occurs within an intellectual environment "enriched by multigenerational interaction, which fosters development of new ideas and encourages risk taking" (Walker et al., 2008). When the dyad mentoring relationship is expanded to a triad, the protégé in turn mentors a new protégé, and all three work together.

The Global Mentoring Process Model provides a framework for describing each of our unique experiences as protégés and/or mentors within both academic and health care systems. Our personal reflections are our contributions to the framework. The experiences of contributing authors in this book provide additional perspectives to enhance nursing's understanding of global mentoring traditions. The model depicts the key factors and mentoring benefits that each individual may or may not have experienced, as each mentoring journey is unique. What follows are our three personal experiences and perspectives on mentoring. It is our hope that in reading the authors' personal reflections, the reader will better understand the described theoretical model, and develop ideas on how it can be used to describe their own personal experiences with mentoring.

Kristina's Reflections

I lived overseas the majority of my childhood and was my older brother's shadow, so I consider him one of my earliest mentors. We attended classes together, from first grade through high school graduation, with an average of a dozen students in each class. This informal mentoring was a daily facet of my life, becoming a life barometer as I reflected on the positives and negatives of our normal sibling verbal exchanges, and I chose which opinions to emulate or discard. I did not realize how much I had depended on hearing my brother's voice in the classroom, serving as a mental backboard to bounce ideas off of, until it was no longer present during my freshman year of college.

During my adolescent years, the innate desire to be understood led me to actively seek out mentoring relationships with teachers whom I considered role models. Although no formal mentoring relationship was established, living in a boarding-school environment allowed observation of key behaviors to determine whether they held true to advice given in the classroom setting. My English teacher's enthusiasm and love of the written word, combined with her respect in listening to children freely express their thoughts, made an impression on my mind and my heart. As a result of this quasi-mentoring experience, I chose to pen poems, attempting to capture thoughts and experiences.

My nursing career and mentoring experiences became intertwined as I progressed along my life's journey. It becomes an exercise of reflection, trying to parse out mentors from friends, or mentors who became friends, and so on. As part of this exercise, I sit here trying out titles, attaching the word "mentor" to this person or another, and then play around with my mental nametags, substituting friend, peer, boss, family, and so on, wanting to be true to the essence of each relationship as I sift through memories. Three things stand out. In my early nursing career my immediate supervisor was a key mentor (Jakubik, 2008). It was a reciprocal mentoring relationship in that we each respected the professionalism of the other and bounced nursing ideas off one another in the quest to perfect our nursing unit. Although reciprocal and of importance, this mentoring relationship was limited in scope to the nursing profession and limited to the time of that nursing unit interaction.

My most memorable mentoring experiences occurred during my PhD nursing program. One faculty member was formally assigned as my mentor and provided insight into being a successful nursing scholar. Having similar life views, her encouragement during my first year of the program bolstered my will to persist with this educational endeavor until its completion. I also had a second mentor during my PhD nursing program. This mentoring relationship has been unique in that it has both formal and informal elements and is a reciprocal mentoring relationship that has evolved over time into a foreseeable lifelong mentoring relationship and friendship. This mentoring relationship differs from a formally established one, as it was a serendipitous outcome of an informal debate over a multitude of topics. Both my mentor and I sought out the mentoring relationship, which is similar to the research findings by

Anibas et al. (2009), and our mentor-protégé relationship then became formalized. The uniqueness of this mentoring experience is that we do not operate with a set of objectives desired from a mentoring experience. Instead, the ground rule established has been to meet on a monthly basis in an atmosphere of trust, with freedom to discuss whichever topic I bring forward. This freedom of expression has resulted in a perfect willingness to debate, which has sharpened my intellect, enhanced my self-confidence, and provided me with an array of career insights. In many ways, this mentoring experience has been one of the highlights of my PhD academic experience. In fact, I am now a mentor, which adheres to Huybrecht et al.'s (2011) finding that students who have had mentors guide their professional growth may in turn mentor others.

Other faculty members also served as informal mentors, which emphasizes the view that each person needs a cadre of mentors, not just one mentor. Because we are multifaceted individuals, one mentor alone cannot meet our varied mentoring needs. Just as my brother was once a life barometer, my husband is now my constant mentor, extrapolating today's happenings and trends, always envisioning a future for me full of potential and career advancement. My husband is the perfect mentor, watching out for my well-being, knowing me better than I know myself at times, always willing to support me by giving advice or standing resolute on a direction he believes will be in my best interest.

Susan's Reflections

A mentor to me is someone who provides support, challenges me, and takes me out of my comfort zone to help me grow. I grew up in a loving, close-knit family in which I was allowed to grow into the person I am today. I credit my parents and my grandparents for always being there to guide me. My grandmother was my first mentor, and she guided me and gave me the confidence to learn to read and know that I could do anything I wanted. She encouraged my creativity and allowed me to think uniquely. She taught me what it meant to care first for myself and for others.

When I was in college and studying to become a nurse, one of my first mentors taught me more than how to wash my hands and give an injection; she taught me that I was capable of being a great nurse (Anibas et al., 2009). Later in school, another informal mentor helped guide me toward my love of caring for pregnant women and infants. Both these faculty members showed me trust and support, similar to Anibas et al's (2009) study suggesting novice faculty need to learn these traits.

In the years that followed, while I worked as a nurse caring for laboring women, receiving my MS and then teaching nursing students, there was a lull in having a significant mentor. I had individuals who provided guidance but were only involved for a short time or only on one project. As time passed, I became the mentor for several nursing students, nurse interns, and new managers. Because I was the mentor, I did not have or feel that I needed anyone to provide support or challenge me. The only person who pushed me during this time was my husband. When I needed extra encouragement, he was there to offer the support and the challenge that I needed to believe that I could accomplish this new goal. When the opportunity arose to attend a new PhD program late in my life, it was my husband who said, "Go and do it!"

When I started the PhD in nursing program, I was assigned a mentor in a formal mentoring program. I met with the person once, and, because it was a new program, we were asked to evaluate the program on how to get the most from a mentor. I decided that I did not need a mentor and would be able to progress with the support I had. I think that I had been a mentor for so long that I did not see the value of having my own mentor. After being in the program for a year, three things happened. First, I formed a close bond with the cohort of students; over the years, we became peer mentors and later mentors to other students as they entered the program. Second, I realized that if I were to succeed and grow, I needed a mentor to guide me and provide support and challenge, as in Jakubik's (2008) study indicating that even mentors with time limitations assisted protégés in being successful. This mentor encouraged me and offered me opportunities to work with other scholars and to practice my research and writing skills. This was a different type of mentoring than I had experienced before, and it continues now after graduation, although the relationship has progressed more to a give-and-take relationship where we each bring something different to the forum, providing a mutual and productive working relationship in which we mentor each other. Third, I found that I needed more than one mentor and so sought a team of mentors when I became a graduate research assistant. The team provided mentoring in research and writing style that I continue to rely on.

What is happening now in my mentoring cycle is that I am once again a mentor, but I approach mentoring with a different perspective. The mentoring structure that I am personally involved in is cascade mentoring (Walker et al., 2008), because it helps me benefit the science of nursing. As I learn from my mentors, I then pass this knowledge on to my protégé(s). Mentoring involves more than teaching, support, and encouragement. It is about the relationship and what it brings to the mentor and to the protégé.

Mary Lou's Reflections

Although I never had a formal mentor as I journeyed from a small town in Nebraska to Kansas, Texas, Mexico, Puerto Rico, Arkansas, and back to Texas, I often found myself in need. Following graduation from high school, I traveled to another small town in Kansas, where I enrolled in a nursing educational program in a Mennonite hospital where the majority of instructors were deaconesses who had devoted themselves and their careers to Christian service. Although I had worked briefly in a Mennonite hospital during my high schools days in Nebraska, the constant immersion experience of living, studying, working, worshipping (chapel required), celebrating, and mourning with them was new for me and one that required much guidance and emotional support.

From Kansas, I went to Texas to continue working toward a bachelor of science in nursing, where I was first exposed to both the "cowboy culture" and persons of Hispanic origin. After my first year of study, I accepted the opportunity to volunteer in a hospital in central Mexico (Aguascalientes, which translates as "hot water"). I was lost without any knowledge of Spanish, cultural customs, and local health care practices. Indeed I found myself in hot water more times than not! Again, I needed emotional support, guidance, knowledge, and role modeling (Gibson & Heartfield, 2005). After spending a second summer in Mexico, I graduated and headed off to Puerto Rico to study nurse-midwifery. By this time, I had taken Spanish classes and, upon landing in San Juan, was ready to begin coursework in a second language. In an area with still different cultural traditions and a variation of the language and expressions, I immediately recognized the need for even more support, role modeling, knowledge, and guidance (Jakubik, 2008; Jakubik et al., 2011; McLaughlin, 2010). With the guidance of faculty, fellow classmates, and colleagues I met within the community, I survived, graduated, and returned to Mexico, where I spent 3 years in nurse-midwifery practice before returning to Texas. It was in Puerto Rico where I experienced what I have since labeled as "rigorous but not ruthless" guidance from professional nurses and faculty who were committed to helping me succeed (without offending too many along the way).

In Mexico, I encountered more "guiding hands." As the only American nurse in the hospital, I depended heavily on support from the nurses, the nurse aides, and the hospital physician to help me learn what to do and what not to do. For instance, I could not believe that I was expected to pierce baby girls' ears when they were dressed to go home! (It was part of their layette and a cultural custom.) A Mexican colleague demonstrated the steps of the procedure twice: once on a baby and then once on me! In this instance, she shared her knowledge and provided emotional support (McLaughlin, 2010).

Back in the United States, in master's and then doctoral programs in nursing, I encountered faculty and classmates whom I now consider to be informal mentors (Davidhizar, 1988) who welcomed me into new academic adventures and challenges and yet more new cultures with differing expectations. Having arrived in Pittsburgh in the middle of the academic year, I experienced emotional support both from classmates who had already completed part of the master's program and from faculty who guided and advised me as I tried to establish networks and fulfill the academic expectations. In Austin, where I pursued my doctoral studies, I was once again the recipient of knowledge shared by recognized scholars and teachers.

I have been a recipient of guiding hands during all my student experiences as well as in my professional roles. As I was guided to practice nursing in Mexico, so have I been guided in my faculty roles, which now span more than 40 years. As a faculty member in Texas in two schools and in Arkansas, I have most valued the tutorage of those who modeled the faculty life (Nies & Troutman-Jordan, 2012).

Were these experiences which I have reflected upon mentoring? If one accepts that mentoring is an "interpersonal process that takes place between a trained, seasoned mentor and a novice protégé" (Mijares, Baxley, & Bond, 2013, p. 27), then perhaps not. None of the individuals about whom I have written were trained, seasoned mentors. Mijares et al. (2013) say that mentoring "entails the provision of emotional support, the sharing of knowledge and experience, role-modeling, and guidance" (p. 27). Using the latter part of this definition of mentoring, then yes, I would conclude that I have been the recipient of informal mentoring the majority of my adult life. This mentoring was found to exist in each culture I encountered within the United States, in Mexico, and in Puerto Rico.

Conclusion

In writing about our experiences, all three of us recognized that essential components of the mentoring relationships were present in each of our separately written personal reflections. These components then became the basis of our Global Mentoring Process Model, which is adapted from Zey's (1991) model. The literature supports these essential components as well as the key factors within the mentoring relationship. It is clear that in our own relationships, this dynamic process is ongoing and meaningful. For example, all three of us experienced supportive mentoring relationships during our doctoral studies (Davidhizar, 1988). Mentors help protégés fulfill their potential (Nelson & Tawiah, 2003) based on the key factors of the mentoring relationship. Writing this book has strengthened our beliefs regarding how mentoring is important not only to our personal and professional development but also to the science of nursing. The contributing authors to this book offer a strong representation of a global perspective on mentoring within nursing.

References

Anibas, M., Brenner, H., & Zorn, C. R. (2009). Experiences described by novice teaching academic staff in baccalaureate nursing education: A focus on mentoring. *Journal of Professional Nursing,* 25(4), 211–217. doi:10.1016/j.profnurs.2009.01.008

Barrett, E. A. (2002). What is nursing science? *Nursing Science Quarterly,* 15(1), 51–60. doi:10.1177/0894318431840201500109

Baxley, S., & Ibitayo, K. (2012). Global mentoring process model. Unpublished model. Copyright 2012 by Copyright Holders.

Davidhizar, R. E. (1988). Mentoring in doctoral education. *Journal of Advanced Nursing, 13,* 775–781. doi:10.1111/j.1365-2648.1988. tb00569.x

Dunham-Taylor, J., Lynn, C. W., Moore, P., McDaniel, S., & Walker, J. K. (2008). What goes around comes around: Improving faculty retention through more effective mentoring. *Journal of Professional Nursing, 24*(6), 337–346. doi:10.1016/j. profnurs.2007.10.013

Elcigil, A., & Sari, H. Y. (2008). Students' opinions about and expectations of effective nursing clinical mentors. *Journal of Nursing Education, 47*(3), 118–122. doi:10.3928/014834-20080301-07

Erdem, F., & Aytemur, J. Ö. (2008). Mentoring—A relationship based on trust: Qualitative research. *Public Personnel Management, 37*(1), 55–65. Retrieved from http://www.ipma-hr.org/node/21487

Fawcett, J. (2012). Thoughts about nursing science and nursing sciencing on the event of the 25th anniversary of nursing science quarterly. *Nursing Science Quarterly, 25*(1), 111–113. doi:10.1177/0894318411429072

Gibson, T., & Heartfield, M. (2005). Mentoring for nurses in general practice: An Australian study. *Journal of Interprofessional Care, 19*(1), 50–62. doi:10.1080/13561820400021742

Grossman, S. C. (2007). *Mentoring in nursing: A dynamic and collaborative process.* New York, NY: Springer.

Grossman, S. C. (2013). *Mentoring in nursing: A dynamic and collaborative process* (2nd ed.). New York, NY: Springer.

Heinrich, K. T., & Oberleitner, M. G. (2012). How a faculty group's peer mentoring of each other's scholarship can enhance retention and recruitment. *Journal of Professional Nursing, 28*(1), 5–12. doi:10.1016/j.profnurs.2011.06.002

Hill, C. W. (2013). *International business: Competing in the global marketplace* (9th ed.). New York, NY: McGraw-Hill/Irwin.

Holmes, D. R., Hodgson, P. K., Simari, R. D., & Nishimura, R. A. (2010). Mentoring: Making the transition from mentee to mentor. *Circulation, 121,* 336–340. doi:10.1161/CIRCULATIONAHA.108.798321

Huybrecht, S., Loeckx, W., Quaeyhaegens, Y., Tobel, D. D., & Mistiaen, W. (2011). Mentoring in nursing education: Perceived characteristics of mentors and the consequences of mentorship. *Nurse Education Today, 31,* 274–278. doi:10.1016/j.nedt.2010.10.022

Jakubik, L. D. (2008). Mentoring beyond the first year: Predictors of mentoring benefits for pediatric staff nurse protégés. *Journal of Pediatric Nursing, 23*(4), 269–281. doi:10.1016/j.pedn2007.05.001

Jakubik, L. D, Eliades, A. B., Gavriloff, C. L., & Weese, M. M. (2011). Nurse mentoring demonstrates a magnetic work environment: Predictors of mentoring benefits among pediatric nurses. *Journal of Pediatric Nursing, 26*(2), 156–164. doi:10.1016/j.pedn.2010.12.006.

Klein, J. (2003). International e-mentoring for a healthy future: The global action network experience. In F. K. Kochan & J. T. Pascarelli (Eds.), *Global perspectives on mentoring: Transforming context, communities, and cultures* (pp. 295–310). Greenwich, CT: Information Age.

McGuire, G. M., & Reger, J. (2003). Feminist co-mentoring: A model for academic professional development. *NWSA Journal, 15*(1), 54–72. Retrieved from http://muse.jhu.edu/journals/nwsa_journal/

McLaughlin, C. (2010). Mentoring: What is it? How do we do it and how do we get more of it? *Health Research and Educational Trust, 45*(3), 871–884. doi:10.1111/j.1475-6773.2010.01090.x

Mijares, L., Baxley, S., & Bond, M. L. (2013). Guiding hands: A concept analysis of mentoring. *Journal of Theory Construction and Testing, (17)*1, 23–28.

Nelson, B. & Tawiah, A. (2003). Insights from two cross-cultural mentoring journeys. In F. K. Kochan & J. T. Pascarelli (Eds.), *Global perspectives on mentoring: Transforming context, communities, and cultures* (pp. 379–398). Greenwich, CT: Information Age.

Nies, M. A., & Troutman-Jordan, M. (2012). Mentoring nurse scientists to meet nursing faculty workforce needs. *Scientific World Journal, 2012,* 1–5. doi:10.1100/2012/345085

Parse, R. R., Barrett, E., Bourgeois, M., Dee, V., Egan, E., Germain, C.,... Wolf, G.. (2000). Nursing theory-guided practice: A definition. *Nursing Science Quarterly, 13*(2), 177. doi:10.1177/08943180022107474

Peterson, D. B., & Hicks, M.D. (1996). *The leader as coach: Strategies for coaching and developing others.* Minneapolis, MN: Personal Decisions.

Walker, G. E., Golde, C. M., Jones, L., Bueschel, A. C., & Hutchings, P. (2008). *The formation of scholars: Rethinking doctoral education for the twenty-first century.* San Francisco: Jossey-Bass.

Zey, M. G. (1991). *The mentor connection.* New Brunswick, NJ: Transaction.

Chapter 2

How Systems Work: Essential Information for Global Mentors

Paulette Burns

Individuals experience systems every day. Such terms as the health care system, the higher education system, the cardiovascular system, and the family system are used in everyday language. Systems are generally recognized and understood by the patterns they exhibit. For example, family systems have many of the same elements but differ greatly in how family members interact with one another, the number and types of family members, the developmental stage of the family, the family communication patterns, goals of the family, family boundaries, values held by the family, and a variety of other variables. Family system A is distinguishable from family system B as different patterns emerge.

As a student, faculty member, or professional nurse, it is important to understand that individuals live, work, and study in systems that affect the individuals and that are affected by the individuals. Understanding systems and how they work increases the likelihood of success in the systems and meeting an individual's educational, professional, and career goals. In addition, a basic understanding of how systems work allows us to more effectively care for patients, families, and communities and to bring about desired changes in ourselves, our workplaces, and our institutions.

This chapter provides a general overview of systems, from the mechanistic worldview and general systems theory (GST) to the more current worldview of complexity theory focusing primarily on complex adaptive systems (CASs) and how they differ from one another, organizations as CASs, navigation of the organizational system, and tips for "fitting into" the CAS.

Why Is a Discussion of Systems Important in a Book About Global Mentoring?

Recognizing and understanding the systems in which an individual is embedded has the potential for opportunities for self-organization that lead to self-emergence or growth, adaptation, and success. Generally, a nurse is involved in many systems simultaneously: self, family, nursing unit or educational program, university or health care agency, health care system or higher education system, community, and the nation or multiple nations. These complex systems interact in ways that affect individuals daily in their positions and roles. Using the lens of systems thinking helps an individual view the system from a broad perspective that includes seeing overall structures, patterns, cycles, and emergence rather than only specific, often disconnected, events. It helps provide a more accurate picture of reality so that a person can work within the system to achieve desired organizational results. This positive feedback to the system then increases the likelihood that individual desired outcomes will be achieved.

Systems are important to discuss in a book about mentoring because individuals entering a new system or performing in a new role in a new system can benefit from a mentoring relationship. Generally, a person who functions as a mentor is one who understands and has successfully navigated the system or role the mentee is beginning. The mentor can fulfill the roles of system coach and guide as the mentee learns the system patterns and ways of behaving in the system to increase likelihood of success in the system. The mentor-mentee relationship provides opportunities for emergence and growth for both individuals.

For example, a newly licensed registered nurse in a first job position is learning to embody and act as a registered nurse while learning about the multiple systems in the overall hospital system that must interact to achieve safe, quality patient care. Generally there is an orientation to the system, but recognition of the need for more intense and longer education and mentoring has been recognized. Consequently, many new nurse residency programs have emerged with mentoring of the new nurse as a major component.

Overview of Systems Thinking

Mechanistic Worldview

Newton's laws of physics provided the foundation for the mechanistic, reductionist science that emerged in the eighteenth century. The Newtonian worldview "considers that all things are equal to, but not more than, the sum of their parts and thus can be somewhat cleanly divided into those parts. Think of an engine that can be divided into gears, cams, and other metal parts. . . . It assumes that all systems are structured like and behave like machines" (Lindberg & Lindberg, 2008, p. 30). Thus the phrases "mechanistic" and "functions like clockwork" have permeated our worldviews in education and health care continuing through today. The same authors further state that the dominant research methods used in reductionist science focus on cause and effect, with the effect being influenced by only a limited number of variables, using quantitative measurement, for the purpose of prediction and control. The objective, controlled scientific method has served society well with new discoveries that have led to the potential for a healthier and higher quality of life. However, this is only one perspective and does not allow for advancing understanding of more holistic challenges.

General Systems Theory

General systems theory (GST), an interdisciplinary school with multiple thought leaders, is proposed in the 1968 book by biologist Ludwig von Bertalanffy, *General System Theory: Foundations, Development, Applications*. He observed many parallels among different disciplines and hoped to unify the study of many disciplines through identification of a GST. A major contribution of the theory is the advancement of holism, a reaction to the mechanistic worldview.

Bertalanffy incorporated ideas about holism that are central to the systems thinking of German philosopher Georg Wilhelm Friedrich Hegel, who stated that the whole was greater than the sum of its parts. A major tenet of GST is the idea that systems consist of a number of interrelated and interconnected parts that, once put together, make the behavior of the whole different and distinct from the behavior of its individual parts. In other words, we cannot understand the behavior of the whole by studying the behavior of its various components (Skyttner, 2006).

Many and varied definitions of a system exist. Skyttner (2006, p. 57) states, "An often used common sense definition is the following: 'A system is a set of interacting units or elements that form an integrated whole intended to perform some function'. Reduced to everyday language we can express it as any structure that exhibits order, pattern and purpose. This in turn implies some constancy over time." GST can be further understood by examining the elements and definitions of a system (Kast & Rosenzweig, 1972, p. 450, which are identified in Table 2.1 with examples provided by Burns.

TABLE 2.1 Major Elements of GST

ELEMENT	DEFINITION/ DESCRIPTION	EXAMPLE(S)
Open to environment	Open systems take in energy from the environment, allowing growth and change over time.	Some open systems are humans, families, communities, hospitals, and universities.
Teleology or purpose	Behavior in systems is teleological or purposeful. The system has one or more goals.	Goals of a university generally include student learning, discovery of new knowledge, and dissemination of new knowledge.
Interrelated subsystems	The behavior of the whole is greater than the sum of its parts; thus the focus on the relationships between the parts is primary in understanding the system.	A university has several academic units as well as others, such as student affairs, budget and finance, communications and marketing, and research, that interact to meet university goals.

ELEMENT	DEFINITION/ DESCRIPTION	EXAMPLE(S)
Input-transformation-output process	A system is in a constant process of taking inputs and transforming them into outputs. The inputs are acquired from the environment, and the outputs go back into the environment in a constant exchange.	Human breathing requires the intake of oxygen from the environment, processing the oxygen within the lungs and throughout the body, and breathing out carbon dioxide into the environment.
Feedback	Feedback allows a system to attain its desired or steady state. There are two types of feedback loops: Negative or positive information on which the system reacts is one that is after the fact; the other is anticipatory and called feed forward control. The system uses feedback to take corrective actions.	A grade that a student receives on a test is negative feedback if it is evaluated as a poor grade. If it is evaluated as a desired grade, then it is considered positive feedback. Adjusting a planned route prior to embarking on it based on traffic patterns is an example of feed forward.
Homeostasis	The ability of a system to achieve a state of dynamic equilibrium maximizes its chances of survival and growth. This state may or may not be the state from which the system initially starts.	The heart's return to normal functioning after a heart attack exemplifies dynamic equilibrium.
Equifinality	This is the ability of a system to attain the same final result from many different approaches.	The nursing education system includes many avenues leading to initial licensure, such as ADN, BSN, 2nd degree accelerated BSN, and alternate entry MSN programs.

continues

TABLE 2.1 Continued

ELEMENT	DEFINITION/ DESCRIPTION	EXAMPLE(S)
Boundary	The line or point where a system or subsystem can be differentiated from its environment or from other subsystems. It can be rigid, permeable, or some point in between. Systems or subsystems will engage in boundary tending.	Boundaries are discernible between the nursing unit and the hospital; the academic department of nursing and the university; the person and the environment.

Complexity Theory, Particularly Complex Adaptive Systems

Health care has become increasingly specialized in the 20th and 21st centuries, while health and health outcomes have become increasingly more difficult to predict and control. For example, the problems of obesity, chronic illnesses, and mental health are not problems that can be addressed using a linear approach, but rather require a framework that takes into account the complexity of such problems.

Complexity science began to emerge in the 1980s and is changing our approaches to science in profound ways. According to Lindberg and Lindberg (2008), complexity science is not a single theory, but rather an interdisciplinary field that recognizes multiple theoretical frameworks including but not limited to such theories as chaos theory, nonlinear dynamics, and complex responsive processes. Complexity theory focuses on complex adaptive systems (CASs), or those systems that are "made up of many interconnected, interdependent, adaptive, and diverse elements" (p. 33). Further understanding of CASs is found in Plsek's (2001, pp. 313–314) outline of the major properties of CAS examples (see Table 2.2).

TABLE 2.2 Properties of Complex Adaptive Systems

ELEMENT	DEFINITION/ DESCRIPTION	EXAMPLE(S)
Adaptable	The elements of the system can change themselves.	Antibiotic-resistant organisms Anyone who learns
Simple rules	Complex outcomes can emerge from a few simple rules locally applied.	CPR guidelines Course grades (author)
Nonlinearity	Small changes can have large effects.	A union-organizing effort that emerges based on a rumor
Emergent behavior, novelty	Continual creativity is a natural state of the system.	Ideas that spring up in the mind
Not predictable in detail	Forecasting is inherently an inexact, yet bounded, art.	Weather forecasting
Inherent order	Systems can be orderly even without central control. Self-organization is the key idea in complexity science.	Termites build the largest structures on Earth when compared with the height of the builders without the guidance of a CEO termite
Context and embeddedness	Systems exist within systems, and this connection matters.	The linking of global stock markets such that if the currency of Thailand falls, the U.S. stock market reacts
Co-evolution	A CAS moves forward through constant tension and balance. Tension, paradox, uncertainty, and anxiety are healthy in a CAS.	The destructive yet essential nature of fires for a healthy, mature forest

A Comparison of General Systems Theory and Complex Adaptive Systems

GST and CASs share similarities but also differ in unique and important ways. CASs build on GST but find GST limited to certain types of systems. Complexity theory focuses on CASs but does not assume that all systems are complex adaptive ones. Both theories propose that energy is taken into the system from the environment, crosses the system boundary, is transformed by the system processes, and then is exported into the environment as outcomes. Notable differences include the cyclical nature of GST and the return to equilibrium, whereas CASs are based on the notion of chaos and adaptation, with adaptation being most likely when near the edge of chaos. CASs exhibit the property of emergence (toward self-organization and adaptation) rather than entropy (increasing disorder and finally death); and instead of seeking homeostasis, as in GST, CASs focus on adaptation and evolution through the processes of self-organization. Because CASs are dynamic and composed of numerous interconnected, interdependent, adaptive, diverse elements, they move closer to chaos and resultant emergence when confronted with challenges. Due to the nonlinearity and nonhierarchical nature of CASs, small changes in one part of the system can bring about large changes in the whole system.

Differences are reflected in the discussion by organizational theorist Stacey (1996), who describes GST as appropriate when there is a high degree of certainty as to outcomes from actions and a high degree of agreement among the people involved in taking the actions. The example he uses is a surgical team doing routine gallbladder surgery. The team brings knowledge and skill about the certainty of procedures that will lead to a positive outcome, and the team members agree on each other's roles and actions so that the surgery and the outcome are predictable. Other issues that have little or no certainty and little or no agreement on actions could be said to be operating in the zone of chaos, one example being a riot in the streets. Or, the health care of victims and their families who experience an unprecedented trauma such as 9/11. Other issues exist in a zone of complexity in which only a modest level of certainty and agreement emerge, such as the debates over providing health care coverage for the uninsured in the United States or managing health care for a population with multiple comorbidities.

Organizations as Complex Adaptive Systems

The contemporary worldview of organizations generally recognizes organizations as CASs, rather than the mechanistic worldview of systems that includes prediction and control, or GST where equilibrium is the goal. As the health care system in the United States evolves with little predictability and high levels of uncertainty, it is organizing in ways that allow new entities to emerge, such as and so-called minute clinics for primary care in high-density shopping markets. Organizations are subject to external and internal influences of interdependent, diverse subsystems that require adaptation and flexibility. The clinical nurse leader is an example of a new nursing role developed in response to the increasing specialization in care units. The role is envisioned as one that will decrease fragmentation of care and increase patient safety and quality care, while lowering costs.

According to Lipmanowicz, chair of the Plexus Institute, organizations are most adaptive and creative when four elements are in place: "rich interactions among the agents in the system; agents [who] are free to self-organize rather than be directed all the time; constant feedback about what is happening; and small changes [that] have a big impact on the system, as those changes ripple through the system and build a critical mass for major change" (Lindberg & Lindberg, 2008, p. 152).

Navigation of the Organizational System

Accepting a new position or role in a health care agency or university or beginning a new degree program is often accompanied by feelings of being overwhelmed or lost (perhaps close to the zone of chaos?) as the individual enters a CAS. For example, a nurse practitioner who has been working for several years providing excellent care with confidence and competence in a health care system completes a nursing doctoral program. The new degree prepares this individual to lead research, and the system expects research products that contribute to the purpose of the system. This new perspective requires the doctoral-prepared nurse to participate in the system in new ways. Having a nurse researcher as a mentor in the organization or external to the organization has the potential to create new insights and actions as the information flow about the nurse researcher role is enhanced for the mentee nurse researcher.

To increase the likelihood of success in navigating the new system, it is important to ask several questions so as to better understand the system. Axelrod and Cohen (2000) provide an extensive list of questions for consideration when using complexity theory in a particular CAS. A few are listed in Table 2.3, with examples reflecting the organizational embeddedness of the individual.

TABLE 2.3 System Assessment

ORGANIZATIONAL SYSTEM QUESTIONS	CLUES	EXAMPLE(S)
Purpose and main function of organization	Mission, vision, and value statements Consider coexisting purposes.	To educate students; to provide health care to the population; to survive as a system; to provide jobs to the community
Philosophy and values of the organization	Written materials about the organization Do the workings of the organization reflect the stated philosophy and values? What are the outcomes that reflect operationalization of the values?	Organization's stated support of the faculty-student relationship belied by high class sizes and faculty-student ratios that allow little time for such interaction outside class
Inputs to the organization	Job opportunities; who/what needs the goods or services of the organization Who/what does the organization need to do its work and create its outputs?	Faculty, students, staff, revenue, technology, regulations

ORGANIZATIONAL SYSTEM QUESTIONS	CLUES	EXAMPLE(S)
Outputs of the organization	Which goods and/or services have been produced? What are by-products of producing the goods and services?	Graduates with degrees and credentials, research findings, effects of salaries on the local economy
Agents (generally people) and what they do	Organizational chart that displays scope of responsibility and span of control of system agents What are the connections between and among agents?	Faculty, administrators, librarians, campus police
Rules of thumb, routines, norms (may be unstated or stated)	Policy, procedures, handbooks, orientation materials, colleagues, observations	Teaching assignments and schedules, expected performance of new faculty or students
Tools and resources agents use to do the work of the system	Artifacts, information, other agents, technology, expertise needed to do the work of the system	Library, writing center, human resources, textbooks, statisticians
Populations of agents (who can learn from whom so that new ideas emerge?)	Committees or task forces across units with like agents as well as different agents	Faculty senate composed of faculty across the university, dean's committee
Which criteria of success does the system use?	Objectives of the organization	Pass rates on state board exams, graduation rates, tenure, profit/loss statements
What is rewarded in the system?	Celebrations recognizing agents, promotions, public announcements	Awards for teaching or research, tenure, cooperation, salary increases, increased responsibility with or without title

TIPS (Thoughts, Ideas, Possible Strategies)

Relationships and interactions are primary areas of focus in a CAS to achieve the desired outcomes for the organization and for the individuals involved. It is essential to build networks of reciprocal interaction that foster trust and cooperation. One way to do this is to promote the informal associations that provide the basis of social capital. For example, as a young faculty member new to academia and the faculty role, I experienced my first clinical teaching day on a medical-surgical floor with 10 students in a hospital and a course new to me. I had been hired in the middle of the semester due to an unexpected faculty vacancy. The day was filled with challenging patient care and student learning situations. I had only an inkling of what the students' competencies were from previous courses and what they were to focus on in the current course. I was feeling on the edge of chaos, lacking in confidence, and questioning my abilities. A senior faculty invited me to coffee to talk over the day. That was the beginning of our mentor-mentee relationship as she listened and offered her acceptance and understanding. We agreed to meet several times during the semester and each time she listened, shared information, and helped me clarify and work through identified challenges. She was instrumental to my understanding of the department of nursing as a system that interacted with the university system and was acted upon by the university system. I have been in academia many years, and still use many of the lessons learned in that first mentoring relationship that allowed me to be a successful educator. Other examples of building reciprocal interaction include organizing a study group, inviting a colleague for lunch, or volunteering for a system committee. Put yourself in situations that will likely lead to development of relationships, such as visiting the lounge for coffee, keeping your door open so that others know they can interact with you, and sitting by different people at meetings so that you get to know more individuals and they get to know you. Dense social ties facilitate information sharing, understanding how things work through others, and reputation building. These are all essential components in establishing a foundation for trust in a complex organization. Identify individuals in the system who hold expertise about its various aspects, and develop working relationships with these people. For example, a new nursing faculty member who will teach primarily in a prelicensure nursing program needs to understand the overall degree program to understand the focus and breadth of the courses to teach. Establishing a good working relationship with the chair of the nursing curriculum committee is vital to implementing the most appropriate courses.

Following or staying near another agent (preceptor, mentor, and colleague) allows you to "learn the ropes" as well as meet the people this agent knows, which increases your own connectivity. At a minimum, a new agent in a system should have access to another agent from whom to learn the general workings of the organization and/or the role to increase the chances of successfully meeting the organization's outcomes. The American Association of Colleges of Nursing has a new dean mentoring program. An experienced dean agrees to mentor a new dean for the purposes of socialization to the dean's role, leadership development, and networking opportunities. The relationship is described as providing mutual benefit, indicating the CAS represented by the relationship has the potential for innovation and emergence of new ideas and strategies for each dean (AACN, 2013).

Another strategy is "legitimate peripheral participation" (Lave & Wagner, 1991), such as participating in hospital rounds, internships, and fellowships. This lets you see how an expert individual works but also allows access to social interactions of the system expert. Nursing students have opportunities to participate in clinical internships. One example is an oncology nursing summer internship program between Texas Christian University and the University of Texas Southwestern Medical Center, Simmons Cancer Center. Students work with the interprofessional oncology team in providing care to cancer patients and their families. The nationally recognized program has successfully recruited new graduate nurses to the field of oncology nursing as a career choice. Oncology care across systems exemplifies a CAS, and the internship experience allows students to participate as agents in meeting the goals of patient care.

If the system does not have a frequent, regular mechanism for feedback in place for new agents or agents with new roles, then ask for regular feedback from an agent in the system whom you trust and who will tell you the truth about your performance, such as your mentor. Regular, frequent feedback allows alterations in the individual subsystem and more optimum functioning in light of system expectations, whether stated or unstated.

Understanding yourself as a CAS is important to function at the highest levels possible on a regular basis. This understanding relates to self-care, self-reflection, and personal growth. Human beings live in a complex world with multiple stressors and opportunities on a daily basis. Caring for yourself through mindful attention to healthy patterns of eating, sleeping, exercise, and management of stressors is important to function well in the organizational system. Cultivating sensitivity to self and others through self-reflection, awareness, and mindfulness daily allows you to understand yourself more fully. Hernandez (2009) is the author of a self-care model for nurses based on Watson's theory of caring (2005). Included in the model are the concepts and behaviors of compassion, awareness, reflection, intentionality, nonjudgmental attachment, and gratitude. Deep understanding of self and of self in relation to others enhances the opportunities for positive interactions and connectivity and a greater chance of system improvement and personal growth.

Within a CAS, it is important to remember that a small change in one part of the system has the possibility of effecting a change in the larger system. This small change could be the change in interaction patterns that occurs because of an individual's self-reflection and choice of new responses. This principle provides great opportunities for seeking new answers to old problems through individual leadership. It is important to remember that the individual brings many valuable inputs to the organization, with the possibility of transforming the organization and the individual. For example, an undergraduate nursing student completed a clinical placement at the local homeless shelter. During her experience, she noticed that there were a lot of people who volunteered to provide services or food, but few talked with or established relationships with the homeless people in the shelter. Understanding that positive human relationships and interactions are foundational to health, she decided to start visiting the homeless people on Lancaster Avenue each Saturday. After a few months, several other students joined her. She petitioned the university and received approval of a new student organization, "Love on Lancaster" which is now in its third year of operation. Every Saturday, the organization members visit homeless people on Lancaster just to talk and build relationships. The student has transformed perspectives about and interactions with homeless people through her leadership in the university.

Swenson and Sims (2012) report that nonhierarchical methodologies based in complexity science can be used to create opportunities for thinking and acting in new ways in organizations. Liberating structures (LS), a concept developed by Lipmanowicz and McCandless (2012, p. 1), are defined as "twenty-five (and growing) easy-to-learn, adaptable methods that make it quick and simple for groups of people of any size to radically change how they interact and work together, and thus how they address issues, solve problems and develop opportunities." One example of a liberating structure is "Drawing Together." The purpose of the activity is to use nonverbal expressions to uncover hidden knowledge and reveal insights that cannot always be understood through words. The activity uses symbols and combinations of symbols to tell the story about the journey of working on a challenge or project (McCandless & Lipmanowicz, 2012, p.1). Swenson and Sims (2012) describe several methods and give examples of how they have been used in a school of nursing. Any of these methods can be applied to any organizational system.

Conclusion

Complexity theory, particularly in relation to CASs, is changing our worldviews and approaches to challenges. The nurse who recognizes and understands this can work within the complexity framework to achieve desired organizational outputs; make a difference for students, patients, families, and communities; and increase the likelihood of achieving desired personal and professional goals.

References

American Association of Colleges of Nursing (2013). New Dean Mentoring Program. Retrieved from http://www.aacn.nche.edu/membership/new-dean-mentoring-program.

Axelrod, R., & Cohen, M. (2000). *Harnessing complexity.* New York, NY: Basic Books.

Hernandez, G. (2009). The HeART of self-C.A.R.I.N.G.: A journey to becoming an optimal healing presence to ourselves and our patients. *Creative Nursing, 15*(3), 129–133.

Kast, F., & Rosenzweig, J. (1972). General systems theory: Applications for organization and management. *Academy of Management Journal, 4*(15), 447–465.

Lave, J., & Wenger, E. (1991). Situated learning: Legitimate peripheral participation. New York, NY: Cambridge University Press.

Lindberg, C., & Lindberg, C. (2008). Nurses take note: A primer on complexity science. In C. Lindberg, S. Nash, & C. Lindberg (Eds.), *On the edge: Nursing in the age of complexity* (pp. 23–48). Bordentown, NJ: PlexusPress, www.PlexusInstitute.org.

Lipmanowicz, H., & McCandless, K. (2012). Frequently asked questions on Liberating Structures. Retrieved from http://c.ymcdn.com/sites/www.plexusinstitute.org/resource/resmgr/liberatingstructures.pdf

McCandless, K., & Lipmanowicz, H. (2012). Liberating Structures: Including and Unleashing Everyone. Retrieved from http://www.liberatingstructures.com/20-drawing-together/

Plsek, P. (2001). Appendix B: Redesigning health care with insights from the science of complex adaptive systems. In Institute of Medicine (Ed.), *Crossing the quality chasm: A new health system for the 21st century* (pp. 309–322). Washington, D.C.: National Academies Press.

Skyttner, L. (2006). *General systems theory: Problems, perspectives, practice* (2nd ed.). River Edge, NJ: World Scientific. Retrieved from http://site.ebrary.com/lib/tculibrary/Doc?id=10201182&ppg=69

Swenson, M., & Sims, S. (2012). Reflective ways of working together: Using liberating structures. In G. Sherwood & S. Horton-Deutsch (Eds.), *Reflective practice: Transforming education and improving outcomes* (pp. 229–244). Indianapolis, IN: Sigma Theta Tau International.

Stacey, R. D. (1996). *Complexity and creativity in organizations.* San Francisco, CA: Berrett-Koehler.

Watson, J. (2005). *Caring science as sacred science.* Philadelphia, PA: F. A. Davis.

Chapter 3
Challenges of the Educational System to Students: A Faculty Perspective

Susan M. Baxley and Kristina S. Ibitayo

Mentoring fosters professional growth (Nettleton & Bray, 2008), so protégés seek multiple mentors as they work in different settings over the course of their educations and careers (Grossman, 2013). Formal mentoring occurs in established mentoring programs with assigned mentors, whereas informal mentoring meets specific needs of the protégé and is nonassigned (Grossman, 2013). In addition, protégés may seek other mentoring activities based upon their varied needs (Grossman, 2013). The educational system is one of many systems described by Paulette Burns in Chapter 2 in which individuals function each day. Mentoring in educational systems is both formal and informal in structure, as informal mentoring occurs within everyday life (Bell & Treleaven, 2011). Mentoring also occurs at different levels based upon the developmental needs of the protégés (Lester, Hannah, Harms,

Vogelgesang, & Avolio, 2011). Individuals have different mentoring needs based upon personal characteristics, age, and where they are in their nursing educations, and the quality of the mentoring relationship is also affected by the mentor's and protégé's personal characteristics, age, and frequency of interactions (Murphy, 2011). To mentor effectively, a mentor needs to assess a protégé's knowledge, cognitive ability, desire for a mentor, and voiced needs. Mentors want to see their protégés achieve their nursing education and career goals; however, the protégés must take the initiative to establish these goals and convey them to their mentors. The mentors or protégés may initiate contact, but both parties need to work to develop and maintain the mentoring relationship. The actual demographic similarities are not as important for a quality mentoring relationship, whereas a mentor and protégé's perception of their similarities makes a difference (de Janasz, Ensher, & Heun, 2008; Turban, Dougherty, & Lee, 2002). Another necessary component of the mentoring relationship is a mentor's skill in listening to the protégé's "future goals, desires, and personal aspirations" (Evans & Forbes, 2012, p. 397).

The basis of a mentoring relationship is mutual trust, which has three factors: the mentor's ability or characteristics needed by the protégé, the mentor's benevolence toward the protégé, and the mentor's perception of the protégé's integrity (Berg, Tsai, Ferguson, & Louie, 2012). Mentors and protégés must exhibit a propensity to trust to begin building a relationship, and this trust in the mentoring relationship grows with each perceived risk and action taken (Berg et al., 2012). A successful outcome of set goals is dependent on this mutual trust (Berg et al., 2012). The concepts of loyalty, prestige, and protection are related to the concept of trust. Loyalty occurs when both mentor and protégé trust each other and believe in the mentoring relationship. A protégé may obtain prestige when working with a mentor who is a recognized figure in the profession of nursing. Conversely, some may also bestow prestige on the mentor when they acknowledge the contributions the mentor has made in helping the protégé achieve educational and professional goals.

The needs of protégés change over time from having one or more senior mentors to using peer mentors and forming a mentoring network (Balmer, D'Alessandro, Risko, & Gusic, 2011). In a formal mentoring program, both mentor and protégé bear the responsibility for initiating the mentoring relationship; however, the protégé is responsible for communicating professional needs and goals for continued growth (Balmer et al., 2011). In contrast, peer mentoring provides a structure for collaborative efforts and ongoing support (Balmer et al., 2011). Co-mentoring uses mantras such as: "No one can get there alone," which exemplifies co-mentoring's non-competitive and safe environment structure, allowing protégés the freedom to take emotional and intellectual risks (Jipson & Paley, 2000, p. 39).

Challenges to Students Within the Educational System

Students face many challenges related to finances, technology, and their environments as they first enter the educational system or return for further studies and degrees. For mentors to understand the challenges of nursing students, they must be aware of financial issues their protégés may face, such as decreased funding for nursing education and the need to seek outside employment while studying. Students may face technological challenges, as the delivery of nursing education continues to change and adapt to the use of available technological advances in the various levels of nursing education (Davis, Davis, & Williams, 2010). The U.S. nursing educational system will become obsolete if it does not utilize this technology (Davis et al. 2010). The educational system needs to adapt to current technology to succeed academically, and all levels of nursing students need to be competent in this technologically savvy world. Many students who are seeking nursing degrees through online programs live in cities, states, or countries far away from the home university. Mentoring needs to adjust to this change in technology as well by including such options as e-mentoring, texting, and video-based conferencing. Additional challenges for nursing students may include the lack of a supportive educational environment in their homes.

Challenges for Bachelor of Science in Nursing Students

Students who are pursuing their bachelor of science in nursing (BSN) degrees face varied challenges, including different educational expectations at the university level, where they need to demonstrate self-initiative and motivation. Compared to students from other disciplines, nursing students are more motivated by extrinsic rewards (Dockery & Barns, 2005). All registered nurses (RN) who graduated in 2005 or later from their initial nursing programs had an average age of 31 years (Health Resources and Services Administration [HRSA], 2010). At an average age of 28, RNs with BSN degrees or higher were 5 years younger than graduates with an initial associate degree in nursing (ADN) or a hospital-based diploma program (HRSA). Older students often approach learning in a more multidimensional way compared to younger students, for whom learning takes place in the context of real-life scenarios and learning by doing (Bye, Pushkar, & Conway, 2007).

Funding a nursing education is a challenge for most nursing students regardless of the degree program. In the 2008 national sample of RNs in the United States, 42.7% of nursing students used family resources to fund their initial education toward becoming RNs, while 30.5% received funding from their jobs in a health-related field, and 29.3% received federally assisted loans (HRSA, 2010).

Educational systems may be challenged to meet the needs of different age groups, which have varied learning expectations and needs. Generation X (people born between 1965 and 1981; Elwood, 2009) and Millennials (people born between 1982 and 2001) are technologically oriented and may prefer receiving educational materials in a digital format (Evans & Forbes, 2012). In contrast, nursing faculty and administration, who are predominantly from the Mature (people born between 1900 and 1945) and Baby Boomer (people born between 1946 and 1964) generations, may be challenged in adapting to new technologies, educational formats, and new ways of communicating with their younger student populations (Evans & Forbes, 2012). In addition, age differences between mentors and protégés may present a challenge.

A unique challenge to BSN students is that they typically do not yet have a career and therefore are more concerned with graduating from their nursing programs than focusing on long-term career goals. They have short-term perspectives, and their mentoring relationships tend to reflect this orientation. Mentoring relationships with BSN students may be more hierarchical rather than collaborative, especially with faculty members. Based on the authors' observations and experiences, peer mentoring is also used by these students as they continuously seek input from peers in a collaborative relationship.

Challenges for Registered Nurse to Bachelor of Science in Nursing Students

According to a study of students in an accelerated second-degree nursing program, the students were attracted to a career in nursing because of the RN shortage and the continued future workforce demand for RNs (Raines, 2010).

In 2008, RNs with ADNs accounted for 45.4% of all RNs with an initial degree in nursing; diploma nurses accounted for 20.4%, and 34.2% had BSNs or higher degrees (HRSA, 2010). It is important to note that since 1980, the educational system has moved away from diploma programs to ADN and BSN programs (HRSA, 2010). RN-to-BSN students may exhibit some of the same characteristics as the generic BSN students, but they also face additional challenges. RN-to-BSN students come from different educational systems and may have already been in the workforce for a number of years, so their readiness to learn needs to be sparked. These learning needs differ from those of other students, as they approach their educations with knowledge based on their clinical experiences; at the same time, these students' knowledge, experiences, and skills are valuable contributions to the learning community (Raines, 2010). In contrast, traditional BSN students may have had limited prior formal clinical training. Before receiving their initial nursing education, 67.2% of RNs (in all degree programs) worked in a health-related field, the majority as nursing aides or assistants (HRSA, 2010).

RN-to-BSN students need to focus on acquiring leadership knowledge, enhancing writing skills, utilizing research, and understanding the scientific reasoning for nursing practice. Nursing faculty may be of the same generation as these students, which may affect their learning environments and any mentoring relationships. Typically, a major portion of this educational program may be offered online, which presents challenges for learning and mentoring. An example noted by the authors is that mentoring of RN-to-BSN students often occurs in the workplace rather than within the academic setting.

Challenges for Master of Science in Nursing Students

Education in a master of science in nursing (MSN) program is based on a foundation of theoretical and empirical knowledge. Beginning MSN students face the challenge of bridging the gap between their undergraduate and graduate studies, requiring that they spend their time effectively producing scholarly products (Abba et al., 1997; Weil, 2001). The decision to seek an MSN degree requires that students devote time learning nursing theory and how to improve patient care by applying theoretical and empirical knowledge. They enter the MSN program with a desire to advance their nursing careers in either leadership, education, or in clinical specialties. An example of a challenge is that these students need to adjust their thinking and learning approach to one with a theoretical perspective.

In the clinical setting, nurse practitioners (NPs) serve as mentors for NP students, socializing them into the advanced practice nurse (APN) role (Hayes, 1998). The mentor commits to a mentoring relationship, which has a longer duration than if the person is serving as a clinical preceptor, and ultimately the mentor contributes to the NP student's perception of self-efficacy (Hayes, 1998).

A unique challenge for MSN students is in transitioning to the APN role and receiving acceptance from peers in this new role. The authors have noted that often while in the midst of their nursing programs, these students may not receive peer support from those not pursuing advanced education. Peers in their working environment may ask MSN students whether they believe themselves to be better than others or why they need to obtain advanced degrees. MSN students need to adjust their thinking and approach in the clinical setting so that it is in line with their newly acquired knowledge. Informal peer mentoring is used frequently, as those with similar educational goals can communicate easier with others due to a similar understanding of adjustments needed in their new roles. There is a need to establish meaningful long-distance relationships, as these students begin to understand the need for long-term guidance and mentoring in fulfilling their varied goals. As nurses complete their MSN programs it is important for them to stay in touch with peers, because experiences and knowledge differ from place to place. Technology and e-mentoring strategies assist in maintaining these long-distance relationships (Byrne & Keefe, 2002). E-mentoring helps mentors connect with their protégés via electronic conversations, vocational guidance, and role-modeling (Rowland, 2012).

Challenges for Doctoral Students

The first challenge for doctoral students is deciding which doctoral program best matches their career goals. The doctor of nursing practice (DNP) degree focuses on clinical practice, whereas the doctor of philosophy (PhD) degree focuses on nursing research (Loomis, Willard, and Cohen, 2006). The doctor of nursing science (DNSc, DNS, DSN) graduate will function as a nurse scientist with expertise in clinical phenomena, the investigative skills of a researcher, and the leadership skills for influencing health care systems. Accelerated programs are increasing in popularity, providing an option to proceed from the BSN to the PhD or the DNP.

Doctoral students may be mid-career and in senior leadership positions and now face the challenge of being a student with sustained scholarly critique while juggling many personal and professional time commitments (Jackson & Cleary, 2011). A major challenge for doctoral students is the length of time elapsed (15 years on average) between graduation with a BSN and graduation with a doctorate (Davis et al., 2010; IOM, 2011). Doctoral nursing students are generally older (age 45–47) compared with other fields (age 33; Cohen, 2011). This may be due to the high number of women in the profession delaying their education because of childbirth and family obligations (Cohen, 2011) or because of "a culture that promotes obtaining clinical expertise prior to continuing graduate education" (IOM, p. 196). Current admission criteria now call for a license to practice nursing in most programs in the United States. Many mid-career doctoral students have mortgages, families, and the related financial obligations (Jackson & Cleary, 2011). Independent-research and critical-thinking skills are fostered in doctoral programs, but the integration of these elements while dealing with everyday life commitments remains a challenge (Jackson & Cleary, 2011). Students who seek the doctoral experience from an accelerated program may or may not face some of the same issues as the mid-career students, depending on when they choose to pursue their degree.

Half of all doctoral students who begin a program never complete their degrees because of financial needs, difficulties with academic preparation, professional development, and lack of mentoring (Holley & Caldwell, 2012). The mentoring program may be formal or informal. One proposed method for obtaining expert mentorship of short-term duration during dissertation studies is through an international collaborative doctorate (Ketefian, Davidson, Daly, Chang, & Srisuphan, 2005). The international collaborative doctorate provides a unique way of networking with experts around the world on global health issues and policy. E-mentoring may also be a part of the mentoring structure used (Rowland, 2012).

The biggest difference between male and female doctoral students in a mentoring relationship is the female students' need for acceptance and confirmation (Bell-Ellison & Dedrick, 2008). In one study, 83% of women perceived that 20% of time in their mentoring relationship was spent on social aspects, while only 60% of men experienced this (Luckhaupt et al., 2005). Additionally, 50% of women believed that gender congruity affected their social professional boundaries, compared to only 12% of men (Luckhaupt et al., 2005). These gender differences need to be accounted for in mentoring relationships.

Doctor of Philosophy students

PhD students have the challenge of recognizing that their research interests may change as they progress in their programs because of refined thinking and new knowledge. They face the challenge of staying true to the passion that brought them into the programs and becoming comfortable with constructive criticism about their research to develop the best research proposals. PhD nursing students face the distinctive challenge of needing faculty mentors with the same research interests (Ketefian et al., 2005). An initial challenge for PhD students is recognizing that although they bring a clinical perspective to their mentoring relationships, the faculty members generally bring a theoretical perspective (Mullen, 2000). They may begin to develop a collaborative relationship when each party recognizes key strengths in the other (Mullen, 2000). An example of a challenge PhD students may face is envisioning themselves as scholars and nurse scientists. Mentoring activities can occur wherever there is a pursuit of scientific inquiry, by transferring knowledge, mentoring research activities, and developing research partnerships (Byrne & Keefe, 2002). The "development of nursing science is the foundation for the growth of the nursing discipline and profession" (Byrne & Keefe, 2002, p. 392).

Doctorate of Nursing Practice students

DNP students face many of the same challenges that PhD students face, such as funding their educations and final projects (Swider et al., 2009). DNP students have the added challenge of developing clear goals and outcomes for their career trajectories. An example of a unique challenge for DNP students is obtaining mentors with DNP degrees. There is some confusion within the nursing community regarding the value of the DNP to the nursing profession (Swider et al., 2009). APNs with DNP degrees can use this credential in the clinical setting but should not use the title "doctor" in the clinical setting without clearly indicating that they are not physicians (Texas Constitution and Statutes, 1999).

Challenges for International Students

To better assist the increasing ethnically diverse U.S. patient population, educational systems need to provide an environment that helps international students succeed. Mentoring is one strategy that nursing faculty members can use to promote the retention of a diverse racial and ethnic student population (Wilson, Andrews, and Leners, 2006). Relational mentoring strategies include communicating, developing professional leadership skills, building confidence, and seeking support (Wilson, Andrews, & Leners, 2006).

Culturally diverse students may need a multicontextual approach to learning, as they perceive the world around them differently and interpret and communicate meaning according to their cultural backgrounds and communication (verbal, nonverbal, associations, etc.) modes (Giddens, 2008).

Challenges for international students include language and cultural barriers, feelings of nonacceptance and cultural isolation, difficulty interpreting instructor cues, financial burdens, lack of orientation to the academic setting, and lack of mentors (Holley & Caldwell, 2012; Starr, 2009). International students who speak English as a second language may face additional difficulties in their nursing educations (Starr, 2009).

Although these students' different cultural beliefs, values, and practices bring richness to the nursing education environment, these same factors may also present a challenge in both the classroom and clinical settings (Starr, 2009).

International students who lack experience in active self-directed learning may memorize facts and expect to be given all information, so faculty members need to redirect international students to interpret facts in light of their own cultures (Starr, 2009). An example of a challenge is that some cultures view faculty as authority figures, and international students may face communication barriers due to feeling unable to communicate freely with faculty.

International students who are just beginning their practice (e.g., BSN students) must be explicitly directed to actively communicate the patients' needs and desires to health team members to truly function as patient advocates. The authors have noted that some of these communication difficulties in not speaking openly to team members may be due to internal cultural desires to respect and please authority figures.

Getting the Most From the Relationship: What a Mentor Can Do for You

Mentoring relationships in which faculty mentors serve as true mentors are usually voluntary in nature, with the mentor freely committing to guiding the protégé (Byrne & Keefe, 2002). Alumni can be used as mentors for students in formal mentoring programs (Sword, Byrne, Drummond-Young, Harmer, & Rush, 2002). Students benefit from this mentoring relationship as learning opportunities and resources are presented to them. Mentors benefit from this relationship as they reconnect with the educational system and nursing profession. In the course of mentoring activities with alumni, the science of nursing is made real to the student rather than just theoretical (Sword et al., 2002).

Protégés seek mentors at different educational or professional phases, depending on their goals, so each mentor sought and each mentoring relationship will be different from another dyad. At the beginning of a mentoring relationship, both mentor and protégé need to understand where each is coming from and the expectations each person has for the relationship. During each mentoring session, goals need to be established regarding what the mentor and protégé expect, and at the conclusion of each session, clear statements need to be formulated regarding how to achieve the goals, including the type of assistance the mentor can provide. In mentoring, the mentor helps the protégé achieve long-term solutions, whereas coaching (a term often confused with mentoring) is a short-term process that occurs on the job and may even be a onetime interaction in response to a question (Theodore, 2012).

Mentors help protégés set goals and understand why they want to achieve these goals. Outcomes need to be clarified at the onset of a mentoring relationship. The Ultimate Success Formula is a six-step process by which knowing the reasons participants set their goals helps them develop a plan, take action, know what they are achieving, and consistently evaluate their progress so that modifications can be made to obtain the desired goals (Eng, 2012).

Strategies for mentors include giving practical guidance, establishing ethical and trusting relationships with their protégés, encouraging communication, promoting engagement with students and faculty, sharing feasible projects, promoting accountability, establishing timelines, reflecting on student experiences, providing opportunities to improve writing skills, maintaining regular feedback, and supporting dissemination of results (Jackson & Cleary, 2011). Mentors can also share their personal experiences on how protégés can be successful in their studies while managing their time commitments.

THINGS A MENTOR CAN DO FOR A PROTÉGÉ

- *Assess the desire for a mentoring relationship, get to know each other, build trust, set goals, and keep the relationship focused on the protégé's desired outcomes (Hart, 2012).*

- *Connect the protégé to the mentor's professional network and provide opportunities to expand their own network.*

- *Help the protégé understand the system, the organizational culture, and the behavioral expectations necessary to attain the protégé's goals.*

- *Help explore options without providing final solutions (Hart, 2012).*

continues

- *Assist the protégé in assessing personal strengths and weaknesses (Hart, 2012).*

- *Offer expertise in a selected area.*

- *Provide protection and a buffer to discrimination by guiding the protégé to see potential threats to the desired outcomes (Hart, 2012).*

- *Maintain awareness of the attitude and practices that are being role-modeled, because the protégé may imitate the mentor while also developing a style that reflects the protégé's personal beliefs and value systems (Hart, 2012).*

- *Inspire the protégé to achieve the stated goals.*

- *Be honest and open to varying views (Hart, 2012).*

- *Offer compassion by providing a supportive environment and ask reflective questions of the protégé so that the student can come up with his or her own solutions.*

- *Demonstrate acceptance of the protégé for the person he or she is (Hart, 2012).*

Responsibilities and Expectations of the Protégé

Although both protégé and mentor agree to establish and develop the mentoring relationship, the protégé has the responsibility to initiate contact with a mentor (McDonald, Mohan, Jackson, Vickers, & Wilkes, 2010), although in a formal program, the mentor may assist the process by contacting the protégé and setting times to meet. It is important for protégés to decide at the onset of mentoring relationships whether they are seeking mentors or coaches, as mentoring assigns ownership and success to the protégés (Theodore, 2012).

Protégés are self-accountable, while the mentors provide guidance. For the mentoring relationship to be successful, protégés must first assess their personal strengths and weaknesses and begin to formulate their goals to best decide which kind of mentor they desire (Kochan & Trimble, 2000). To assess their personal strengths, protégés can use different inventories, such as the Myers-Briggs Type Indicator or the Thomas-Kilmann Conflict Mode Instrument (Kochan & Trimble, 2000).

TIPS FOR PROTÉGÉS

Upper-level students may find the use of reflective journaling useful in assessing their personal achievements, needs, goals, and action plans with timelines for achieving desired goals (Harrington, 2011). Other tips that protégés may use are as follows:

- *Maintain open communication with their mentors on a regular basis (authors).*

- *Share their goals and needs with their mentors (authors).*

- *Be willing to invest in the steps needed to achieve their goals while overcoming perceived obstacles (authors).*

- *Proactively ask for advice from and give feedback to mentors (Hart, 2012).*

- *Be receptive to mentors' advice and feedback (Hart, 2012).*

- *Evaluate the mentoring relationship and terminate the relationship if the protégés' desired outcomes are not met (authors).*

- *Seek the guidance of the program director in a formal mentoring program in terminating the mentoring relationship (authors).*

- *Seek different mentors' expertise when protégés no longer fit with their current mentors and/or their goals change (authors).*

- *Terminate the mentoring relationship with mutual respect and honesty (Hart, 2012).*

Mentoring and Evaluation: Are They Compatible?

Evaluation in mentoring is controversial, as evaluating a protégé falls more within the scope of an adviser's role than a mentor's (Grossman, 2007). The assumption that advisers or role models also serve as mentors has been debated, as has the collective responsibility of faculty for the ethical and professional behavior of their students (Swazey, 2001; Weil, 2001). Evaluation may not be compatible with a collaborative mentoring relationship, as it inserts a hierarchical structure and may impede trust and freedom in communication, which are essential components of a mentoring relationship. Formal evaluation occurs in a coaching context and on more of a short-term basis. Mentoring activities and experiences may occur as a part of an evaluation process to help the protégé reach desired goals, but this situation is different from when a protégé seeks input from a mentor by requesting informal evaluation of progress toward stated goals and objectives (Swazey, 2001; Weil, 2001).

Personal Examples of Mentoring at Different Educational Levels

Throughout the authors' nursing careers, their own mentors exhibited some of these mentoring qualities. They also employed select strategies when mentoring individuals during their different levels of education. This section provides personal examples of mentoring experienced by the authors at different education levels. Sharing these personal experiences may show how mentoring relationships are all different but are similar in that they provide the protégés with people to help them reach their goals. Mentor-protégé relationships must be based on trust and mutual respect, as these experiences demonstrate.

As a BSN student without prior nursing experience, Susan Baxley recalls one mentor as being exceptional because she provided information about the field of obstetrical nursing. By sharing her personal experiences, this mentor inspired Baxley to enter this field of nursing. Her mentor offered her expertise and encouragement as she assessed her personal strengths and weaknesses. After graduation, Baxley used the knowledge provided by her mentor to strengthen her nursing practice and incorporated some of her teaching techniques when teaching obstetrical nursing. Therefore, mentoring can have a lasting influence on a protégé's nursing career and long-term goals.

Kristina Ibitayo offers the perspective of an RN-to-BSN student. Ibitayo earned her BSN degree more than a decade after getting her ADN. Her mentoring needs differed from those of a beginning nurse, because she was already advancing in her nursing career in a charge nurse role. During this time, Ibitayo's nurse manager was an influential mentor who encouraged her to pursue a BSN degree. Her mentor said that some nurses need to soar as eagles and advance their long-term nursing goals by means of advancing their nursing educations. Ibitayo also experienced co-mentoring with this individual as they challenged each other to continually perform at the highest levels of nursing expertise within their separate roles. This informal mentoring relationship resulted in continued advancement for both in their respective nursing careers.

Baxley and Ibitayo pursued MSN degrees for a similar reason: They were in transitional phases of their nursing careers. However, their mentoring relationships during this time were different. Knowing that her lifelong nursing goal included involvement in the global health arena, Ibitayo's mentor explored educational options and motivated her to seek an MSN degree in the administrative track. Her mentor provided compassion and assisted her in redefining her educational focus, helping her decide to drop the MBA portion of the dual-degree program and pursue a PhD after graduating with an MSN.

In comparison, Baxley sought an MSN degree because she knew that she wanted an advanced nursing degree. Because NP programs were not readily available, she took courses in all three MSN tracks (administrative, education, and clinical) to keep her career options open. During Baxley's program, two faculty members assisted her in assessing personal strengths, motivated her to complete the program, assisted her in the clinical setting, and provided her with a new desire to teach.

Interestingly, Baxley and Ibitayo sought doctoral education from the same university, within 1 year of each other. Mary Lou Bond, the other author of this book, served as an informal mentor to both, even before they began PhD studies. Bond's expertise with the Hispanic population and the PhD program's focus on vulnerable populations encouraged Baxley and Ibitayo to apply to the program. At the beginning of the program, they were each assigned a formal mentor, and their mentoring relationships took different paths. Based on their career and scholarship goals, they recognized the need for a formal mentor yet also sought out both informal and peer mentoring relationships. Their formal mentors provided them with mutually trusting relationships, freedom of expression, and supportive environments. Informal mentors were sought for their expertise in applicable areas of knowledge, while peer mentors formed a support network during PhD studies contributing to their success. The majority of these mentoring relationships still continue. Baxley's and Ibitayo's mentors provided them with nurturing environments, which allowed them to explore needed steps and varied solutions for achieving their professional dreams. As protégés, their mentors connected them to their professional networks in different ways.

Mentoring relationships evolve over time. Both Baxley and Ibitayo experienced transitions with their formal mentors, who are now a co-mentor (Baxley) or a friend and advice giver (Ibitayo). Co-mentoring allows for freedom of expression and an exchange of intellectual ideas between peers. Mentors in these relationships also benefit, valuing their protégés' expertise and seeking their input. Each participant inspires the other, providing ideas and opportunities that may not have otherwise been envisioned.

Baxley and Ibitayo realized that they each needed more than one mentor and therefore established additional mentoring relationships with individuals who could best meet those needs. The majority of these mentoring relationships are still in place but have evolved over time into friendships and peer mentoring.

The ways in which Baxley and Ibitayo mentor their own protégés have been influenced by past and current mentoring relationships. Because their mentors exhibited diverse mentoring characteristics, they were each able to develop our own mentoring styles. Mentors should be prepared to adjust their mentoring styles, depending on the protégés' expressed needs and levels of nursing education.

Conclusion

Every mentoring relationship is unique in that protégés have different needs depending on their personal characteristics, educational levels, and short-term and long-term objectives. The personality of mentors and their mentoring styles also contribute to the chemistry of the mentoring relationships, but each mentoring dyad employs a mentoring structure that is mutually beneficial and challenges the protégé to achieve the desired professional aspirations.

Based on the literature, as well as the authors' experiences and thoughts, the protégé is ultimately responsible for the direction and duration of the mentoring relationship, while the mentor's focus is on the protégé and the desired outcomes (Weil, 2001). As with any relationship, mentors may also choose to end the mentoring relationships, especially if they believe they cannot meet the protégés' needs; in this case, they may recommend other mentors who can better meet these needs. In any case, the protégé may not realize the full benefits of a mentoring relationship until years later when she/he reflects on the value of information shared in the mentoring process. A creative environment in a mentoring relationship is based on mutual trust and freedom of communication, where both mentors and protégés benefit from the sharing of ideas and needs (Jipson & Paley, 2000).

References

Abba, I., Ayele, M., Kelly, L., Wheaden-Pugh, T., Wiggs, L., & Wimbuish, S. (1997). Bridging the gap between undergraduate and graduate school. *ABNF Journal, 8*(1), 17–19. Retrieved from www.tuckerpub.com/abnf.htm

Balmer, D., D'Alessandro, D., Risko, W., & Gusic, M. E. (2011). How mentoring relationships evolve: A longitudinal study of academic pediatricians in a physician educator faculty development program. *Journal of Continuing Education in the Health Professions, 31*(2), 81–86. Retrieved from www.jcehp.com/

Bell, A., & Treleaven, L. (2011). Looking for professor right: Mentee selection of mentors in a formal mentoring program. *Higher Education, 61*, 545–561. doi:10.1007/s10734-010-9348-0

Bell-Ellison, B. A., & Dedrick, R. F. (2008). What do doctoral students value in their ideal mentor? *Research in Higher Education, 49*(6), 555–567. doi:10.1007/s11162-008-9085-8

Berg, A., Tsai, J., Ferguson, V., & Louie, B. (October, 2012). *The importance of trust in a research-based undergraduate mentoring program*. Paper session presented at the meeting of 5th Annual Mentoring Conference, Albuquerque, NM.

Bye, D., Pushkar, D., & Conway, M. (2007). Motivation, interest, and positive affect in traditional and nontraditional undergraduate students. *Adult Education Quarterly, 57*(2), 141–158. doi:10.1177/0741713606294235

Byrne, M. W., & Keefe, M. R. (2002). Building research competence in nursing through mentoring. *Journal of Nursing Scholarship, 34*(4), 391–396. doi:10.1111/j.1547-5069.2002.00391.x

Cohen, S. M. (2011). Doctoral persistence and doctoral program completion among nurses. *Nursing Forum, 46* (2), 64-70. doi: 10.1111/j.1744-6198.2011.00212.x

Davis, S. P., Davis, D. D., & Williams, D. D. (2010). Challenges and issues facing the future of nursing education: Implications for ethnic minority faculty and students. *Journal of Cultural Diversity, 17*(4), 122–126. Retrieved from www.tuckerpub.com/jcd.htm

de Janasz, S. C., Ensher, E. A., & Heun, C. (2008). Virtual relationships and real benefits: Using e-mentoring to connect business students with practicing managers. *Mentoring & Tutoring: Partnership in Learning, 16*(4), 394–411. doi:10.1080/13611260802433775

Dockery, A. M., & Barns, A. (2005). Who'd be a nurse? Some evidence on career choice in Australia. *Australian Bulletin of Labour, 31*(4), 350–383. Retrieved from http://espace.library. curtin.edu.au/R/?func=dbin-jump-full&object_id=20894&local_ base=GEN01-ERA02

Elwood, E. (2009). Population bulletin. 20th-century U.S. generations. *Population Reference Bureau, 64*(1). Retrieved from www.prb.org

Eng, D. L. (October, 2012). *Ultimate success formula.* Paper session presented at the meeting of 5th Annual Mentoring Conference, Albuquerque, NM.

Evans, R. R., & Forbes, L. (2012). Mentoring the "net generation": Faculty perspectives in health education. *College Student Journal, 46*(2), 397–404. Retrieved from http://www.projectinnovation.biz/ index.html

Giddens, J. F. (2008). Achieving diversity in nursing through multicontextual learning environments. *Nursing Outlook, 56*(2), 78–83.e71. doi:10.1016/j.outlook.2007.11.003

Grossman, S. C. (2007). *Mentoring in nursing: A dynamic and collaborative process.* New York, NY: Springer.

Grossman, S. C. (2013). *Mentoring in nursing: A dynamic and collaborative process* (2nd ed.). New York, NY: Springer.

Harrington, S. (2011). Mentoring new nurse practitioners to accelerate their development as primary care providers: A literature review. *Journal of the American Academy of Nurse Practitioners, 23*(4), 168–174. doi:10.1111/j.1745-7599.2011.00601.x

Hart, W. (2012). *The seven functions of mentoring.* Center for Creative Leadership. Retrieved from www.ccl.org/leadership/community/mentoringWebinar.aspx

Hayes, E. (1998). Mentoring and self-efficacy for advanced nursing practice: A philosophical approach for nurse practitioner preceptors. *Journal of the American Academy of Nurse Practitioners, 10*(2), 53–57. doi:10.1111/j.1745-7599.1998.tb00495.x

Health Resources and Services Administration (HRSA). (2010). *The registered nurse population: Findings from the 2008 National Sample Survey of Registered Nurses.* Retrieved from bhpr.hrsa.gov/healthforce/resurvey2008.html

Holley, K. A., & Caldwell, M. L. (2012). The challenges of designing and implementing a doctoral student mentoring program. *Innovative Higher Education, 37*(3), 243–253. doi:10.1007/s10755-011-9203-y

Institute of Medicine (2011). *The future of nursing: Leading change, advancing health.* Atlanta, GA: The National Academics Press.

Jackson, D., & Cleary, M. (2011). Practical advice to support mid-career doctoral students in nursing: Some considerations for academic supervisors. *Contemporary Nurse: A Journal for the Australian Nursing Profession, 38*(1), 171–179. doi:10.5172/conu.2011.38.1-2.171

Jipson, J., & Paley, N. (2000). Because no one gets there alone: Collaboration as co-mentoring. *Theory Into Practice, 39*(1), 36–42. doi:10.1207/s15430421tip3901_6

Ketefian, S., Davidson, P., Daly, J., Chang, E., & Srisuphan, W. (2005). Issues and challenges in international doctoral education in nursing. *Nursing and Health Sciences, 7*(3), 150–156. Retrieved from http://onlinelibrary.wiley.com/journal/10.1111/(ISSN)1442-2018

Kochan, F. K., & Trimble, S. B. (2000). From mentoring to co-mentoring: Establishing collaborative relationships. *Theory Into Practice, 39*(1), 20. doi:10.1207/s15430421tip3901_4

Lester, P. B., Hannah, S. T., Harms, P. D., Vogelgesang, G. R., & Avolio, B. J. (2011). Mentoring impact on leader efficiency development: A field experiment. *Academy of Management Learning and Education, 10*(3), 409–429. doi:10.5465/amle.2010.0047

Loomis, J. A., Willard, B., & Cohen, J. (2006). Difficult professional choices: Deciding between the PhD and the DNP in nursing. *Online Journal of Issues in Nursing, 12*(1). doi:10.3912/OJIN.Vol12No1PPT02

Luckhaupt, S. E., Chin, M. H., Mangione, C. M., Phillips, R. S., Bell, D., Leonard, A. C., & Tsevat, J. (2005). Mentorship in academic general internal medicine: Results of a survey of mentors. *Journal of General Internal Medicine, 20*(11), 1014–1018. doi:10.1111/j.1525-1497.2005.215.x

McDonald, G., Mohan, S., Jackson, D., Vickers, M. H., & Wilkes, L. (2010). Continuing connections: The experiences of retired and senior working nurse mentors. *Journal of Clinical Nursing, 19*(23), 3547–3554. doi:10.1111/j.1365-2702.2010.03365.x

Mullen, C. A. (2000). Constructing co-mentoring partnerships: Walkways we must travel. *Theory Into Practice, 39*(1), 4–11. doi:10.1207/s15430421tip3901_2

Murphy, W. M. (2011). From e-mentoring to blended mentoring: Increasing students' developmental initiation and mentors' satisfaction. *Advocacy of Management Learning and Education, 10*(4), 606–622. doi:10.5465/amle.2010.0090

Nettleton, P., & Bray, L. (2008). Current mentorship schemes might be doing our students a disservice. *Nurse Education in Practice, 8*(3), 205–212. doi:10.1016/j.nepr.2007.08.003

Raines, D. A. (2010). What attracts second degree students to a career in nursing? *Online Journal of Issues in Nursing, 16*(1). doi:10.3912/OJIN.Vol16No01PPT03

Rowland, K. N. (2012). E-mentoring: An innovative twist to traditional mentoring. *Journal of Technology Management and Innovation, 7*(1), 229–237. Retrieved from http://www.jotmi.org

Starr, K. (2009). Nursing education challenges: Students with English as an additional language. *Journal of Nursing Education, 48*(9), 478–487. doi:10.3928/01484834-20090610-01

Swazey, J. P. (2001). Graduate students and mentors: The need for divine intervention. Commentary on 'Mentoring: Some ethical considerations' (Weil). *Science and Engineering Ethics, 7*(4), 483–485. Retrieved from http://www.springer.com/social+sciences/applied+ethics/journal/11948

Swider, S. M., Levin, P., Cowell, J., Breakwell, S., Holland, P., & Wallinder, J. (2009). Community/public health nursing practice leaders' views of the doctorate of nursing practice. *Public Health Nursing, 26*(5), 405–411. doi:10.1111/j.1525-1446.2009.00798.x

Sword, W., Byrne, C., Drummond-Young, M., Harmer, M., & Rush, J. (2002). Nursing alumni as student mentors: Nurturing professional growth. *Nurse education today, 22*(5), 427-432. doi:10.1054/nedt.2000.0742

Texas Constitution and Statutes. (1999). Texas Occupations Code. Title 3. Health Professions. Subtitle A. Provisions applying to health professions generally. Chapter 104, Healing art practitioners. Sections 104.003 & 104.004 Healing Art Identification Act. Retrieved from http://www.statutes.legis.state.tx.us/Docs/OCpdf/OC.104.pdf

Theodore, D. (October, 2012). *Mentoring vs. coaching: A manager's guide.* Paper session presented at the meeting of 5th Annual Mentoring Conference, Albuquerque, NM.

Turban, D. B., Dougherty, T. W., & Lee, F. K. (2002). Gender, race, and perceived similarity effects in developmental relationships: The moderating role of relationship duration. *Journal of Vocational Behavior, 61*(2), 240–262. Retrieved from http://www. journals.elsevier.com/journal-of-vocational-behavior/

Weil, V. (2001). Mentoring: Some ethical considerations. *Science and Engineering Ethics, 7*(4), 471–482. Retrived from http://www. springer.com/social+sciences/applied+ethics/journal/11948

Wilson, V. W., Andrews, M., & Leners, D. W. (2006). Mentoring as a strategy for retaining racially and ethnically diverse students in nursing programs. *Journal of Multicultural Nursing and Health (JMCNH), 12*(3), 17–23.

Chapter 4
Challenges of the Educational System to Faculty

David Anthony (Tony) Forrester

Nurses learn to be good nurses by working with other good nurses. Teachers learn to be good teachers by working with other good teachers. Excellent nurse educators achieve excellence by paying attention to excellent mentors and excellent students. Nursing faculty can benefit from effective mentorship by experienced others at every stage of their career.

This chapter addresses the challenges that all nursing faculty members face as they negotiate various systems in higher education. Tips are provided for nursing faculty in general, new nursing faculty who are just getting started and trying to fit into the system and the faculty role one step at a time, seasoned nursing faculty who are striving to be engaged and meet the leadership challenge, nontenure- and tenure-track faculty who are developing themselves as stakeholders, adjunct and clinical faculty who are involved in the academic enterprise, and international faculty who are integrating into the American educational system.

All Nurse Faculty
Understanding the Culture of Your School of Nursing and University

The history and reputation of your school of nursing and its relationship to the community are important factors to assess, both from the perspective of your own career goals and from the perspective of the students you teach. Understanding these factors and the culture of your school of nursing and university is important in developing your overall view of the school and the quality of education you provide (Fitzpatrick & Montgomery, 2006). Remember, the names of the schools of nursing in which you teach will always be listed on your curriculum vitae and will follow you throughout your academic career; make your choices good ones.

Nursing faculty members not only are expected to be familiar with their school of nursing's norms regarding grade reporting, student attendance, academic appeals, and so forth but must develop an understanding of their roles in the school's governance and leadership. Additionally, faculty members must have a working understanding of academic freedom, faculty workload, academic tenure, intellectual property, and possibly even collective bargaining. Much of the information related to these topics is available in published school/university documents, such as faculty bylaws, handbooks, and policy manuals. The American Association of University Professors (AAUP; www.aaup.org) is also an excellent source of information regarding many topics of interest to faculty.

Tips:

- Review the school of nursing's and university's mission, vision, and philosophy statements to ensure congruence with your own mission, vision, and philosophy.

- Review your faculty appointment contract to determine the terms and conditions of your employment, including your workload obligations. Your faculty workload has important implications for your own career planning in meeting the many competing demands of your nursing faculty role (Gerolamo & Roemer, 2011; Hawkins & Fontenot, 2009).

- Review the school of nursing's and university's tables of organization to determine lines of reporting and scope of authority of faculty administrators, instructors, and staff.

- Review the school of nursing's and university's faculty bylaws to understand your role in institutional governance.

- Review all school of nursing and university policies to determine your various responsibilities in carrying out your faculty role.

- Review the criteria for appointment and promotion to academic rank to determine the expectations you must fulfill in achieving excellence in teaching, research/scholarship, and service.

- Review the faculty handbook to understand the rights and privileges of faculty.

- Review the student handbook to understand the rights and privileges of students.

New Faculty: Fitting Into the System and the Faculty Role, One Step at a Time

Getting started in your new role as a faculty member can be daunting. Ideally, you have carefully selected a school of nursing within a university whose mission, vision, and philosophy are consistent with your own. Now it is your responsibility to be proactive in learning about the system you are working in, how you "fit," and how you will participate with others for the mutual benefit of faculty, staff, and students. The nursing faculty role includes many competing demands, such as teaching, practice, and scholarship. A seasoned faculty mentor can help you find balance among these expectations. To get started, several key areas require your attention and participation, including serving on committees, developing your professional network, understanding faculty unionization, identifying resources for faculty development, and understanding legal implications of the faculty role.

Serving on Committees

All nursing faculty members are expected to serve on committees as prescribed by their school of nursing's and university's bylaws. This is how the work of self-governance gets done. Newer, less experienced faculty should probably have minimal involvement during their first 1 to 2 years of employment and focus more on developing their classroom/clinical practicum teaching skills and their scholarship (Fitzpatrick & Montgomery, 2006). As you develop your networking skills, political awareness, and particular areas of interest and talent, you will be wise to invest your energies into committees of particular interest and importance to you and your school. For example, if you are primarily involved in the undergraduate program offerings, you may wish to serve on the undergraduate curriculum committee, which is important in defining, implementing, and evaluating the undergraduate program. Career nursing faculty may later be more interested in serving on the faculty appointment, promotion, and tenure committee, which makes important recommendations to the school's leadership regarding promotion and tenure of nursing faculty.

Tips:

- Make yourself aware of the expectations of your school of nursing and university regarding your membership on and participation in governing committees.

- When deciding which committees to join, seek advice from your mentor(s). An experienced faculty mentor is likely to be helpful in assessing the school's needs, faculty politics, and how you might fit in given your own knowledge and skill mix and in ways that will best benefit your learning in your new faculty role.

- Be selective in choosing committees for involvement to avoid becoming overwhelmed with activities that may interfere with your teaching excellence and/or scholarly productivity.

- Join committees that (1) are interesting to you, (2) will impart new knowledge, (3) will add to your professional credentials and overall credibility as a faculty leader, and (4) are consistent in meeting and advancing your career development goals.

Developing a Professional Network

Professional networking skills are essential to a successful career in higher education in nursing. Successful faculty members create "win-win" collegial partnerships with others both within their institutions and in the international community. Such collaborative partnerships are mutually beneficial and advance both partners' career objectives in their specific specialized areas of teaching, practice, and scholarship. Such partnerships also have the potential to provide tremendous personal and career satisfaction while advancing the nursing profession globally. An experienced faculty mentor will be helpful in guiding you to success in increasing your scope of influence both within your school and university and in the global nursing professional community. Your mentor is likely to encourage you to take on new challenges—activities you perhaps have not thought yourself capable of before. Examples of such challenges may be taking on new leadership responsibilities within your school of nursing, such as serving as a course or level coordinator and participating in, or even chairing, an important standing committee in accordance with your school of nursing's bylaws. Your mentor may encourage you to extend your scope of influence beyond the school of nursing. Running for an office in your chapter of Sigma Theta Tau International, taking on leadership roles on regional or national professional boards, or becoming a reviewer for professional journals are all excellent opportunities to expand you scope of influence in nursing.

Tips:

- Reach out to colleagues to proactively build a supportive network. Ask someone to lunch. Sitting alone in your office and waiting for others to knock on your door is not likely to result in fast friendships.

- Make a conscious effort to develop your networking skills, including remembering the names of people you meet, carrying business cards to share as needed, and being flexible when scheduling meetings.

- Identify and seek out approachable key individuals within your school of nursing and university system with whom you have common teaching, scholarly, and/or practice interests and professional goals.

- Ask others for advice or to read and critique a manuscript. This is flattering to others and communicates professionalism and a desire to establish a mentoring relationship.

- When you identify vacant positions in the table of organization, ask whether you can participate in the selection of an individual to fill that position.

- Develop collaborative relationships that offer mutual benefit for you and your colleagues, while always considering others' career development goals as well as your own.

- Partner with others in your school of nursing, university, and national/international professional/scholarly organizations in teaching, scholarly, and practice activities.

Understanding Faculty Unionization

Although it is perhaps not an essential factor in determining whether you will accept a faculty appointment in a given university, you should determine ahead of time whether faculty members are unionized. If the faculty are represented by a collective bargaining unit, you should become familiar with the details of the union contract, as it affects your terms and conditions of employment.

Tips:

- Determine whether the faculty are unionized and/or whether members are interested in becoming unionized.

- If the faculty are unionized, review all formal union documents, including contracts, letters, etc.

- Develop an understanding of faculty governance and academic freedom in your school.

- Meet with key representatives of the faculty organization to identify and become aware of current issues confronting the faculty and the school of nursing's and university's administration.

Identifying Resources for Faculty Development

Resources for faculty development probably exist both within your school of nursing and within your university. These may include consultation to support your instructional and scholarly development and financial support for continuing your education and attending professional/scholarly conferences.

Tips:

- Work with your mentor(s) to develop a list of immediate (1-year) and long term (5-year) faculty career goals.

- Identify the school of nursing and university resources available to assist you in meeting your career goals.

- If faculty development resources are not available to meet your goals, determine how you might access them individually through outside networking and collaboration, perhaps through a professional or scholarly association like Sigma Theta Tau International.

Understanding Legal Implications of the Faculty Role

It is important to be aware of the legal implications of your faculty role, such as knowing exactly what your position description prescribes for classroom and clinical practicum instruction, clinical agency requirements, and liability insurance coverage. Legal requirements vary widely when providing instruction and clinical supervision for prelicensure nursing students and licensed nurses enrolled in an advanced practice program. You should know about any requirements for students' liability insurance coverage as well as institutional expectations regarding your personal professional liability insurance coverage. A seasoned mentor will be helpful in advising you regarding institutional policies, personal experiences, and perhaps even experiences with legal litigation and how you might avoid it.

Tips:

- Understand your state's nurse practice act so that you have confidence you are teaching students to practice within the statutory authority of a nurse in your jurisdiction.

- Familiarize yourself with the policies of your school of nursing, university, and any collaborating clinical agencies.

- Review your personal professional liability policy very carefully and determine the liability coverage that may be provided by your university to decide whether you have sufficient insurance coverage.

- Make sure that students have obtained all required health clearance and health insurance.

- Discuss the legal implications of being a nursing faculty member with your mentor and other faculty colleagues.

Seasoned Faculty: Being Engaged and Meeting the Leadership Challenge

The National League for Nursing's (NLN's) Nurse Educator Competencies clearly state that nursing educators are expected to "function as change agents and leaders" and use their leadership skills to "envision new realities for preparing graduates for practice in an ever-changing, complex health care environment" (Halstead, 2007, p. 116). Nurse educator leadership development through mentorship and education is strongly advocated for the development of leaders in nursing education who "take risks and face challenges to create environments in which others want to work—leaders who transform nursing education" (Young, Pearsall, Stiles, & Horton-Deutsch, 2011, p. 228).

Fitzpatrick (2010, p. 275) speaks of the "energetic engagement" of nursing faculty and uses the evidence-based model set forth by Kouzes and Posner in *The Leadership Challenge* (2007) in identifying the five key behaviors of nursing faculty leaders: (1) *modeling the way* by creating standards of excellence in nursing education, sharing these standards with peers, and serving as role models of excellence; (2) *inspiring a shared vision* by believing they can still make a difference by engaging others in dreams, generating enthusiasm for the future of nursing education, and engaging others through their work; (3) *challenging the process* by challenging the status quo, taking risks to achieve excellence, learning from mistakes made along the way, and understanding that learning occurs with both success and failure; (4) *enabling others to act* by actively involving others in team building and strengthening each member of the nursing education team, including students who will be the nursing educators and leaders of the future; and (5) *encouraging the heart* by creating opportunities for nursing education team members to share the rewards of success, such as passing rates on National Council Licensure Examination (NCLEX) and certification examinations, and the accomplishments and achievements of graduates and faculty colleagues.

Tips:

- Seek out and carefully choose mentors who can facilitate your faculty leadership development.

- Seek out and be accepting of leadership opportunities within your school of nursing and in your state, national, and international professional networks.

- Continue developing your professional network and expanding your scope of influence through participation in professional/scholarly associations.

- Take informed strategic risks in attempting something new and speaking up. For example, volunteer to serve as a course coordinator, lead an innovative curriculum improvement project, or pursue a leadership role in a regional or national nursing professional organization.

Nontenure-Track and Tenure-Track Faculty: Becoming a Stakeholder in the Academic Enterprise

Academic tenure is the promise of permanent employment and is achieved following a probationary period, usually 6 years. Once tenure is awarded, employment can be terminated only for extraordinary circumstances and financial exigencies (Penn, 2008). Tenure to the university involves a reciprocal responsibility on the part of the university and the faculty member (Billings & Halstead, 2009). As a faculty member, you are expected to remain competent and productive in teaching, research/scholarship, and service while maintaining high standards of professional conduct. Tenure provides you with the protection of greater academic freedom, which is the "freedom . . . to explore new ideas and theories unimpeded" (Whicker, Kronenfield, & Strickland, 1993, p.14). This freedom allows you to freely express your views in the classroom despite any opposing efforts by the government, university administrators, other faculty, students, and others (Billings & Halstead, 2009).

Academic promotion refers to advancement in rank, usually progressing from instructor to assistant, associate, and eventually full professor. Some nursing faculty choose to remain on the nontenure track, content to remain instructors or assistant professors and unconcerned with publishing extensively and advancing to the higher academic ranks of associate or full professor (Fitzpatrick & Montgomery, 2006). It should be pointed out, however, that all nursing faculty are expected to remain competent to teach and current in nursing practice. Additionally, all nurse faculty members are expected to produce at least some published scholarship (Billings & Halstead, 2009), such as evidence-based clinical practice guidelines prescribing best practices at the junior ranks of instructor and assistant professor and original research and scholarship at the senior ranks of associate professor and professor.

The criteria for promotion and achieving academic tenure are closely linked with the overall mission of the school of nursing and university. Teaching-intensive institutions, for example, require that faculty members produce evidence of excellence in teaching with some productivity in scholarship. Academic promotions and the award of tenure in these institutions are based primarily on teaching performance. By contrast, research-intensive institutions expect both teaching and research excellence but likely value research productivity more highly and weigh it more heavily in making decisions regarding academic promotion and tenure.

Understanding the Criteria for Appointment, Promotion, and Tenure

Every school of nursing and university have published guidelines or criteria for faculty appointment, promotion, and tenure. It is important to be aware of these, as they often vary from one university to another and sometimes even between schools within the same university. Senior faculty, faculty administrators, and mentors can help you navigate formal and informal faculty expectations and give advice regarding the coordination of teaching, practice, and scholarly activities to better ensure faculty success.

Tips:

- Review the school of nursing's and university's published mission, vision, and philosophy statements.

- Review the school of nursing's and university's published criteria for appointment, promotion, and tenure.

- Discuss the criteria for appointment, promotion, and tenure with your mentor(s) and faculty colleagues.

- Choose the type of faculty appointment (nontenure track or tenure track) that you find most appealing based on your career goals.

Adjunct and Clinical Faculty: Being Involved

As enrollments in schools of nursing have increased, more and more adjunct and clinical faculty are being employed to meet this demand (Peters & Boylston, 2006). Adjunct nursing faculty members are typically experts in clinical practice who bring up-to-date practice knowledge and skills to the academic setting. Clinical nursing faculty members teach primarily in the clinical practicum setting and may have little or no classroom teaching responsibility. Both adjunct and clinical faculty may be full- or part-time, often have limited contact with members of the full-time faculty, and may not have been educated on their academic roles. It is essential that adjunct and clinical faculty ensure clinical competence, select appropriate clinical assignments, accurately monitor and supervise students' progress, and, when and where possible, engage in scholarly faculty practice.

Ensuring Clinical Competence

Students and clinical agencies have a reasonable expectation that faculty are teaching within their areas of clinical expertise. It is clearly important to avoid teaching in clinical areas outside your area of expertise or in areas in which you are not current in practice. Doing otherwise is inconsistent with the goal of providing quality education and safe patient care. If there is a shortage of nursing faculty to teach in a particular clinical area and you are asked to step into an area in which you do not feel confident, discuss this situation with a trusted mentor and the faculty administrator you report to. This can be an uncomfortable position to be in, and you and your students are likely to benefit from some good advice about how to proceed. In addition to the 12 tips that follow, remember that questioning your clinical teaching assignment should be a collegial, matter of fact, professional conversation. You and your faculty administrator have a shared interest in providing students with a high-quality, safe learning experience while ensuring safe patient care in the clinical practicum environment.

Tips:

- Negotiate with your faculty administrator to teach in clinical areas that are consistent with your area(s) of clinical specialty expertise and greatest experience.

- Decline clinical teaching assignments in areas in which you believe your expertise is insufficient.

- Review basic nursing texts and, time permitting, attend continuing education programs in the content area you are teaching.

- Arrange for an orientation to the clinical site well in advance of student arrival.

- Familiarize yourself with the policies of the clinical agency by reviewing its policy and procedure manuals and any other relevant materials.

- Talk to nurses practicing on the units in which you will be supervising students.

- Report any unsafe practice conditions to the clinical agency and your faculty administrator(s).

- Carefully instruct students regarding their own and others' safety in the clinical setting.

- Insist on a student-faculty ratio that promotes student learning and ensures a safe practice environment—usually a maximum of 8:1 or 10:1.

- Check in with students frequently throughout their clinical practicum experiences.

- Carefully monitor students' progress, focusing especially on students who may be experiencing difficulty in meeting learning objectives or who may be at risk in terms of patient safety.

- Exclude students from the clinical environment who are deemed unsafe in their clinical practice behavior.

Selecting Appropriate Clinical Assignments and Monitoring and Supervising Students' Progress

It is the responsibility of all nursing faculty to accurately assess students' knowledge and readiness to provide safe care for the patient population to which they are assigned. To make clinical practicum assignments that are safe and appropriate, faculty members must be aware of the didactic content students have received and demonstrated competence in through careful, accurate evaluation. An experienced faculty mentor is likely to have insight to offer regarding how you might partner with other faculty who are teaching your students so that you can better keep up with their progress in their programs of study.

Tips:

- Carefully align clinical practicum experiences with course objectives, what students are currently learning in the classroom, and previous courses.

- Ascertain students' knowledge and psychomotor skills during clinical practicum experiences, including pre- and postconferences.

- Monitor staff-patient ratios for potentially unsafe conditions, as they potentially affect student learning and may raise issues of liability.

Understanding the Scholarly Faculty Practice Plan

A scholarly faculty practice plan (FPP) is a formal agreement between a school of nursing and a clinical facility that simultaneously meets the school's mission to provide professional nursing services, education, research/scholarship, and community service (Dracup, 2004; Saxe et al., 2004). Some schools of nursing have scholarly FPPs, while others do not. Whether a school has an FPP is typically related to the school's mission statement. For example, if a school of nursing resides within an academic health sciences university, expert clinical practice, clinically relevant scholarship, and provision of health care to the community are likely to be highly valued. Regardless of the university setting, however, most nursing faculty members benefit their scholarly careers and the quality of their students' instruction by engaging in faculty practice. A scholarly FPP may provide a framework for successfully integrating the teaching, scholarly, and practice expectations of the nursing faculty role.

The purposes of a scholarly FPP are to make the professional nursing services of the school of nursing faculty available to patients, their families, and their communities; make available to all patients, irrespective of place of residence, economic status, or type of need, a uniformly high standard of nursing care; provide nursing students with education in the philosophy, science, and practice of nursing; and generate and report new knowledge through scholarly scientific investigations directed toward improving nursing care and urban health systems (Forrester, O'Keefe, & Torres, 2008).

A scholarly FPP should provide opportunities for professional development of the nursing faculty (e.g., nursing practice, research/scholarship, and teaching skills maintenance/enhancement), enhancement of classroom and clinical practicum instruction for nursing students, generation of faculty and student scholarly outcomes (e.g., scholarly publications and presentations), and generation of revenue for the school and possible salary augmentation for participating faculty members (Forrester et al., 2008).

Funds generated by a scholarly FPP may be used to attract and retain high-quality faculty to teach, do research, and engage in nursing practice; and enable nursing faculty to maintain and enhance their skills as practicing nurses, educators, and researchers/scholars (Forrester et al., 2008). The degree, manner, and number of hours of participation in the FPP are typically matters of negotiation between each participating faculty member and the appropriate faculty administrator, the dean, and the affiliated institution prior to the beginning of the academic year. Each participating faculty member, in collaboration with the appropriate faculty administrator, determines the mutually agreed-upon set of goals and objectives for each contractual year. Participating faculty members should negotiate their contractual agreement between the school of nursing and the affiliated institution so that it clearly specifies the terms and conditions of the faculty practice activity (Forrester et al., 2008).

Tips:

- Determine whether a scholarly FPP is in place in your school of nursing and how it relates to the school's mission.

- Discuss the FPP with your mentor and the key faculty administrator(s) responsible for implementing the plan.

- Determine the implications of your participation in the FPP for your workload, performance evaluation, and compensation.

- If no scholarly FPP is in place, ask about the potential for developing and implementing such a plan.

Challenges of Integrating International Faculty

International nursing faculty members bring value to the school of nursing and university by contributing cultural diversity to the faculty and sharing their own unique experiences and perspectives with their students. Students and tenured or nontenured faculty may serve international faculty as "cultural mentors" by assisting them in gaining an understanding of faculty role expectations as well as generally held social norms in what may be a very unfamiliar cultural environment. It should also be noted that international faculty often provide special assistance to international students by serving as their mentors. Although this may be particularly true when the faculty member and student have a shared country of origin, simply sharing the experience of being an international faculty member and student is likely to enhance the faculty-student mentoring experience.

International faculty members face challenges beyond those of other nursing faculty. Integrating international faculty into nursing's system of higher education often entails difficulties in teaching and research as well as social challenges (Early Career Geoscience Faculty, n.d.). International faculty must adapt to both the "classroom culture" and the "popular culture" while adjusting to teaching in a foreign language, English. International nursing faculty members are also required to produce the same scholarship and publications as their American counterparts.

Challenges in Teaching

The challenges international faculty encounter in teaching include adapting to the U.S. classroom culture, possibly teaching in a foreign language, cultural literacy, and lack of familiarity with the "standard" nursing curriculum.

TIPS for adapting to the U.S. classroom culture

Students in the United States may have different expectations than international faculty regarding appropriate classroom behavior, challenges to authority, and when to ask questions. To adapt to the U.S. classroom culture:

- Talk to your mentor and faculty colleagues about what constitutes "normal" student behavior.

- Visit faculty colleagues' classrooms to observe how they interact with students.
- Be clear when communicating your expectations regarding appropriate classroom behavior, such as collaboration on assignments.

TIPS for teaching in a foreign language

Teaching in a foreign language offers multiple challenges, such as communicating complex thoughts and ideas and making yourself understood to students who may not be familiar with your accent. To become comfortable teaching in a foreign language:

- Take advantage of teaching-related faculty development workshops and programs.
- If available, visit your campus Teaching-Learning Center and inquire about its services. Many teaching-learning centers offer valuable services including workshops or courses designed to help you improve your teaching effectiveness and efficiency as well as other faculty development programs. Additionally, you may find assistance with integrating new technology and innovative evidence-based teaching strategies into your teaching "tool kit."
- Use PowerPoint slides and handout materials to illustrate important points and terminology so that students may more easily follow what you are saying.

TIPS for achieving cultural literacy

If you were not raised in the United States, you may not be familiar with American popular culture. To achieve cultural literacy:

- Engage your students and learn from them by inviting them to come to class a few minutes early for informal conversation about what they like to do outside class.
- Engage your faculty colleagues by participating in school and university social events. Share your experiences and compare them with those of your faculty colleagues.
- Read the newspaper, watch television, and listen to the radio.

TIPS for becoming familiar with the "standard" nursing curriculum

If you were educated outside the United States, you may not be sure what students know when they come into your classroom. To familiarize yourself with the standard nursing curriculum:

- Find out what is taught in prerequisite courses. Talk to faculty colleagues who teach these courses and review their course syllabi.

- Review the requirements for admission into the programs in which you teach.

Challenges in Research

International faculty may encounter additional challenges in conducting research. One such challenge is obtaining research funding.

TIPS for research funding

Some agencies only grant funds to U.S. citizens or permanent residents. To aid your search for funding:

- Discuss grant-funding opportunities with your mentor and your school/university research administrator(s).

- Search out granting agencies that do not have such restrictions, such as the National Science Foundation.

Social Challenges

International nursing faculty may encounter a number of social challenges, such as feeling isolated and distant from friends and family, dealing with racism/ignorance, and establishing healthy working relationships with students.

TIPS for overcoming feelings of isolation

Any faculty member can become lonely as a result of moving to a new location and working long hours. To forge bonds in a new place:

- Host a potluck dinner party for other faculty members with whom you wish to become acquainted.

- Introduce yourself to international faculty and student organizations that may be available at your university.

- Take advantage of inexpensive, sometimes free, technology, such as webcasts, to communicate regularly with friends and family who are far away.

TIPS for dealing with racism/ignorance

You may be fortunate enough to never encounter racism/ignorance, but it is best to be prepared for the possibility in the following ways:

- Reach out to colleagues to proactively build a supportive network. Teach others about your culture and learn about theirs.

- If available, work through your campus office of cultural affairs to create cultural exchanges with faculty colleagues and students.

- Remember that racial hostility and lack of understanding are born of ignorance and have nothing to do with you specifically as a person.

Conclusion

Nursing faculty serve not only as mentors to their students but as mentors to other faculty as well. In turn, all nursing faculty are in need of mentorship throughout their careers. Whether they are new to the faculty role or are seasoned, tenured faculty members with decades of experience, nursing faculty benefit from the experiences and learned wisdom of others around them. A successful faculty career trajectory is best ensured by paying close attention to the behaviors of successful faculty colleagues at every career stage and thoughtfully reflecting on how emulating these behaviors might benefit yourself, students, other faculty members, your school and university, and, ultimately, the global community.

References

Billings, D. M., & Halstead, J. A. (2009). *Teaching in nursing: A guide for faculty*. St. Louis, MO: Saunders Elsevier.

Dracup, K. (2004). Impact of faculty practice on an academic institution's mission and vision. *Nursing Outlook, 52*(4), 174–178.

Early Career Geoscience Faculty: Teaching, Research and Managing Your Career – International Faculty Members. (n.d.). *On the Cutting Edge: An NAGT Professional Development Program for Geoscience Faculty*. Retrieved from http://serc.carleton.edu/NAGTWorkshops/earlycareer/international/index.html.

Fitzpatrick, J. J. (2010). Energetic engagement: The leadership challenge for nurse educators. *Nursing Education Perspectives, 31*(5), 275.

Fitzpatrick, J. J., & Montgomery, K. S. (2006). *Career success strategies for nurse educators*. Philadelphia, PA: F. A. Davis.

Forrester, D. A., O'Keefe, T., & Torres, S. (2008). Professor in residence program: A nursing faculty practice. *Journal of Professional Nursing, 24*(5), 275–280.

Gerolamo, A. M., & Roemer, G. F. (2011). Workload and the nurse faculty shortage: Implications for policy and research. *Nursing Outlook, 59*, 259–265.

Halstead, J. (Ed.). (2007). *Nursing educator competencies: Creating an evidence-based practice for nurse educators*. New York, NY: National League for Nursing.

Hawkins, J. W., & Fontenot, H. (2009). What do you mean you want me to teach, do research, engage in service, and clinical practice? Views from the trenches: The novice, the expert. *Journal of the American Academy of Nurse Practitioners, 21*, 358–361.

Kouzes, J. M., & Posner, B. Z. (2007). *The leadership challenge* (4th ed.). San Francisco, CA: Jossey-Bass.

Penn, B. K. (2008). *Mastering the teaching role: A guide for nurse educators.* Philadelphia, PA: F. A. Davis.

Peters, M. A., & Boylston, M. (2006). Mentoring adjunct faculty: Innovative solutions. *Nurse Educator, 31*(2), 61–64.

Saxe, J. M., Burgel, B. J., Collins-Bride, G. M., Stringari-Murray, A., Dennehy, P., & Holzemer, W. (2004). Strategic planning for UCSF's community health nursing faculty practices. *Nursing Outlook, 52*(4), 179–188.

Whicker, M., Kronenfield, J., & Strickland, R. (1993). *Getting tenure.* Newbury Park, CA: Sage.

Young, P. K., Pearsall, C., Stiles, K. A., & Horton-Deutsch, S. (2011). Becoming a nursing faculty leader. *Nursing Education Perspectives, 32*(4), 222–228.

Chapter 5
Academic Mentoring of Faculty

Roberta K. Olson

The shortage of new registered nurses (RNs) has been documented over time in the nursing literature. The looming shortage of nursing faculty is also becoming a critical issue, as an increasing number of seasoned faculty members are predicted to retire within the next few years (Brendtro & Hegge, 2000; Gwyn, 2011). This chapter describes the importance of mentoring nursing faculty at all stages in their academic careers to provide support, facilitate engagement, promote measurable outcomes, and retain faculty in academia who have the clinical and teaching experience to facilitate student learning. Recruitment and retention of knowledgeable, effective faculty mentors require a multifaceted approach.

The process of mentoring others is an established concept. The key is to be intentional about implementing a process that is tailored for the mentor and protégé to ensure support, learning, and success in the faculty role for the protégé. This chapter describes mentoring at different stages in an academic career, including the responsibilities of the mentor and protégé with support from administration for the process.

Mentoring Structures

Mentorship in nursing education settings provides career enhancement for students, faculty, and administrators. Research studies and anecdotal reports validate that mentor relationships support professional and personal development for both the mentor and protégé. Mentoring leads to professional success and personal satisfaction. The literature discusses the critical nature of faculty shortages and the need to provide mentorship support for newly hired faculty members to retain them in the academic setting (Bland, Taylor, Shollen, Weber-Main, & Mulcahy, 2009; Clark, Alcala-Van Houten, & Perea-Ryan, 2010; Dunham-Taylor, Lynn, Moore, McDaniel, & Walker, 2008; Gwyn, 2011; Sawatzky & Enns, 2009; Slimmer, 2012; Vance & Olson, 1998).

The profession of nursing depends on a community of scholars to conduct research that leads to sound policy decisions, improves access to health care for underserved population groups, and enhances the science of nursing (Bunkers, 2005). Novice nurse educators need to be socialized into their new faculty roles to integrate scholarship into their research, teaching, and service and learn to balance academic priorities. Novice faculty members have excellent clinical skills but need to expand that role by understanding scholarship and facilitating learning in students (Clark et al., 2010; Zimmerman & Yeaworth, 1985). Academic administrators need a broad perspective in their roles. Mentorship facilitates this process for administrators by showing them how to set priorities, bring in consultants for new or difficult areas, and envision the "big" picture (Vance & Olson, 1998).

An attitude of helpfulness from the mentor and the willingness of the protégé to accept useful coaching are essential to achieve expected outcomes in academia. There must be mutual interest, personal relationship "chemistry," and a commitment from the mentor to provide the time and frank advice that is integrated with constant support when the protégé is struggling and feels overwhelmed with the expectations and challenges of a faculty role. Mentoring is not a "new" concept, but it needs focus, nurturing, and continual renewal to provide support and guidance for new and ongoing academicians to remain energized and achieve meaningful outcomes. Dunham-Taylor et al. (2008) provide a helpful activity diagram of mentoring activities for spiraling up with positive mentoring and spiraling down with ineffective or no mentoring.

Spiraling up includes providing enculturation to campus, department, individual courses, and clinical areas; balancing work and personal life; using the wisdom of more experienced faculty; accepting generational diversity; and being willing to share with peers. *Spiraling down* includes forcing individual faculty members to figure things out on their own; encouraging burn-out and personal problems; modeling horizontal hostility; fostering a competitive environment; and fighting generational differences. Figure 5.1 summarizes the essential elements of these processes.

Activity	Spiral Up	Spiral Down
Socialization	Providing enculturation to campus, department, individual course, clinical area	Permitting individual faculty member to discern
Collaboration	Becoming connected as a team; sharpening skills at teamwork	Fostering us versus them mentality; me versus everyone else
Operations orientation	Providing explanations of written/unwritten rules, policies, and procedures	Allowing individual faculty members to discern; tolerating learning by "mistakes as you go"
Validation	Providing feedback and constructive criticism from peers, leaders, and students to improve teaching skill and self-esteem	Allowing physical and social isolation; allowing ineffective teaching/advising to occur/recur
Expectations	Balancing work and personal life	Encouraging burn-out and personal problems
Transformation	Monitoring and encouraging role transition (novice to expert); encouraging use of talents, skills, and strengths to create future nursing leaders	Modeling horizontal hostility, professional hazing, "eating the young"; fostering competitive environment
Reputation/Inspiration	Illustrating appropriate behavior for academic and local community; providing positive motivation	Modeling and/or allowing inappropriate behavior detrimental to academia, nursing, and local community; dampening spirit and excitement
Documentation	Facilitating development of professional portfolio; teaching importance of documenting interaction with students	Allowing promotion credits to lag; fostering laissez-faire attitude with students
Generation	Using wisdom of more experienced faculty; generation diversity; willingness to share with peers	Recreating the wheel; fighting generational differences
Perfection	Modeling and encouraging scholarship, service, research, and teaching effectively; does not require perfection	Obstructing career advancement in scholarship, service, teaching, and research; requiring perfection

FIGURE 5.1

Mentoring activities: Spiraling up with positive mentoring and spiraling down with ineffective or no mentoring. Dunham-Taylor et al, (2008), p. 341. Used with permission of Elsevier and Dr. Dunham-Taylor.

Various Mentoring Models

Various types of mentoring models are described in the literature (Advisory Board Company, 2009; Campinha-Bacote, 2010; Daloz, 1986; Dalton, Thompson, & Price, 1977; Dunham-Taylor et al., 2008; Heinrich & Oberleitner, 2012; Vance, 2011; Vance & Olson, 1998). A mentoring model can be either formal or informal, and a mentor in a formal or informal relationship can be a seasoned or peer faculty member. A formal model is intentional and includes an organized plan for the provision of guidance over time. An informal model is more "happenstance" and occurs when a faculty member seeks and receives information to solve an immediate situation in more of a "one-dose" exposure without "boosters." The multifaceted variables for successful outcomes include the culture of the academic setting, needs of the faculty at various career stages, and mentors and administrators who understand the mentoring process.

How to Mentor Faculty: Who Mentors Whom?

This section focuses on common behaviors and responsibilities for both mentor and protégé plus stages along a career trajectory for the novice, the mid-career professional seeking tenure and promotion, and the experienced professional ready for post-tenure opportunities. The key elements are the trust and respect in the relationship between the mentor and protégé. The ideal pattern is to have the mentor and protégé mutually select each other and set up a plan. The usual, practical method is to begin with an assignment of a seasoned faculty member to a novice faculty member. Each mentor-protégé relationship is unique because of the objectives that are identified for the development of the protégé. However, the goal of each relationship is to foster the learning curve of the protégé to understanding the role, early engagement, and productive outcomes. Common behaviors and responsibilities for the mentor and protégé are described in Table 5.1.

TABLE 5.1 Mentor and Protégé Common Behaviors and Responsibilities

MENTOR BEHAVIORS/ RESPONSIBILITIES	PROTÉGÉ BEHAVIORS/ RESPONSIBILITIES

• Supportive encouragement and honest feedback to protégé
 • Validation of knowledge and work output
 • Guide for behavioral changes that may be needed
 • Availability for regular or informal meetings
    • Establishes regular meeting times
    • Takes to lunch and meetings
    • Introduces protégé to others; opens doors for collaborative relationships
 • Personal characteristics
    • Maturity
    • Emotional intelligence (Goleman, 1995)
    • Security in own knowledge
    • In developmental stage of generativity (Erikson, 1963); interest and ability to give to the next generation
	• Receptive to guidance and coaching from mentor
	 • Follows through with suggestions from mentor
	    • Sets aside time for regular meetings with mentor
	    • Journals experiences and questions
	    • Completes format for tenure and promotion data
	 • Personal characteristics
	    • Security in own knowledge, but acknowledgment of the need to learn and ask questions
	    • Intellectual curiosity

RESPONSIBILITIES FOR BOTH MENTOR AND PROTÉGÉ

- Mutually establish expectations
- Develop a professional development plan (PDP) for 3 and 5 years for the protégé (see Table 5.3 template)
  - Stretch goals for 3 and 5 years to prepare for tenure and promotion or, in the case of a term master's-prepared faculty member, plans to complete doctoral preparation
  - Establish measurable objectives for annual work plan
- Personal characteristics
  - Effective time-management and organizational skills
  - Relationship that is built on trust and respect
  - Frankness in discussions to create an optimum learning environment

Available Opportunities for Mentors and Protégés: Who, When, Why, and How

Mentoring Novice Faculty

Development of a professional or a scholarly trajectory can be done at any stage of an individual's career. It is essential that novice faculty members understand the importance of being mentored and seek examples that provide guidance. One such example is described by Banks (2012), who outlines strategies for faculty to balance work-related goals along with other priorities in their lives. A list of questions provides guidelines related to decisions for a scholarly trajectory. Garand et al. (2010) have developed a tool, the professional development plan (PDP), to guide junior faculty in their progression toward promotion and tenure. Faculty on the tenure track reported that the tool was a helpful guide for focusing their scholarship outcomes. Martin and Hodge (2011) describe how senior faculty worked with master's-prepared faculty to mentor them during various research projects. These mentored partnerships provided professional development, mastery of new skills, and support from the department to engage in the role of faculty. Anibas, Brenner, and Zorn (2009) outline a program for teaching academic staff (TAS) developed by their university to prepare expert staff nurses to teach clinical sections of undergraduate students by mentoring them (described in Table 5.2 as "Clinical Assistants").

Hegge et al. (2010) describe a clinical academic partnership (CAP) with one university and one Magnet facility. The CAP project paired two staff nurses with one faculty member to supervise eight students on a nursing unit. Each CAP nurse supervised two students, and the faculty member supervised four students and served as a mentor. The CAP nurses enrolled in a three-credit graduate course designed to provide them with information on supervising and evaluating nursing student learning. The five-module online course integrated (1) the art of nursing in the teaching-learning process, (2) discussion of principles of leadership, (3) application of the principles of teaching and learning in the clinical setting, (4) factors within the diverse clinical environment that influence teaching and learning, and (5) application of principles of evaluation. CAP staff nurses reported that their confidence and competence as clinical assistants with undergraduate students increased with their learning from this course. Since this partnership began in 2006, a majority of CAP nurses have enrolled in graduate studies and completed their master of science in nurse education programs.

Mentoring on the Tenure Track

Typically, a tenure-track faculty member (often holding the title assistant professor) has a time period of 6 years during which to achieve tenure and promotion to the rank of associate professor. There is ongoing discussion about the value of tenure for the individual and the university, but at this time, the tenure process is alive in most universities, and a faculty member on the tenure track must understand the need to prepare a well-documented dossier when the due date is reached. It is essential that, when the tenure track begins, the assistant professor have a 6 year plan in place to be successful in achieving tenure. No magic potions or processes can be applied to make this process happen; it is dependent on the faculty member's ability to develop a clear plan with stretch goals and annual achievable, measureable objectives. The plan requires insight and guidance from a seasoned and tenured associate professor or professor. The work requires that the assistant professor be engaged, intentional, and focused and balance demanding priorities.

Jacelon, Zucker, Staccarini, and Henneman (2003) provide information on how peer mentoring was successful at their school in assisting new assistant professors achieve tenure and promotion. The authors cite the values of developing relationships among diverse faculty, creating opportunities for collaboration on research projects, and developing camaraderie among faculty throughout the university. Garand et al. (2010) have developed a tool to assist junior faculty in their progress toward tenure and promotion. Testimonies from junior faculty who have used the tool to measure their progress indicate that the tool is extremely helpful. Dunham-Taylor et al. (2008) emphasize the importance of ongoing mentoring for new and seasoned faculty. Mentoring is the most influential process for successful faculty development and retention.

Mentoring Post-Tenure

Table 5.4 lists organizations that provide leadership programs with an emphasis on being mentored. These opportunities can be considered while faculty are on the tenure track, but they are particularly appropriate for tenured associate professors who aspire to become department chairs and deans. Table 5.2 describes different responsibilities of the mentor and the protégé with regard to (a) pursuing post-tenure opportunities; (b) completing tenure-track work; (c) being term doctorally prepared; (d) being term master's prepared; (e) serving as an adjunct; and (f) working as a clinical assistant.

TABLE 5.2 Mentor and Protégé Responsibilities Vary for Tenured, Tenure-Track, Term, Adjunct Faculty, and Clinical Assistants

FACULTY TITLE	DIFFERENT RESPONSIBILITIES	
	MENTOR	PROTÉGÉ
Tenured, seasoned faculty	• Recognized leader in the profession • Excellent teacher, researcher • Engaged in similar research or teaching as the protégé • Guides continued publication of data-based manuscripts	Tenured Associate Professor • 3- to 5-year professional development plan (PDP) for continued productivity • Post-tenure review plan • Serve as leader in regional or national professional organization • Earn national recognition for expertise in area of research, teaching, or service • Explore opportunities for further leadership development (see Table 5.4).
Tenure track	• Steers PDP development • Guides increasing evidence of protégé's scholarship, teaching, and service productivity while creating a focus and balance in the workload	Assistant Professor • 3- to 5-6 year PDP to achieve tenure; review tool in Garand et al. (2010) • Narrowed focus of scholarship in research, teaching, and service • Increased leadership responsibilities within college and university

FACULTY TITLE	DIFFERENT RESPONSIBILITIES	
	MENTOR	PROTÉGÉ
	• Facilitates selection of external mentor to assist with research focus	
Term DNP or Phd-prepared Regular 9-month full- or part-time	• Matches with seasoned faculty in same clinical or teaching area • Oversees area of expertise and need as defined by the college	Instructor, Lecturer, or Senior Lecturer • Prepares 3- to 5-year plan for academic career progression • Provides selected course or clinical content as needed with favorable assessment by students and mentor
Term MS-prepared	• Matches with seasoned faculty in same clinical or teaching area • Guides development of plan for career progression • Performs peer observation in classroom and clinical • Provides support and feedback in classroom and clinical teaching • Facilitates inclusion on scholarship projects within the college	Instructor with an MS in Nursing Education • Prepares 3- to 5-year plan for: • Evidence of successful teaching strategies in classroom and clinical • Completion of doctoral degree • Certification as Nurse Educator • Experience with presentations, manuscript writing, and member of scholarship project(s) • Serves as committee member within the college
Adjunct	• Helps administrator or course coordinator orient to expectations	Adjunct part-time who is recognized for expertise • Provides selected course content as needed with favorable assessment by students and mentor

continues

TABLE 5.2 Continued

FACULTY TITLE	DIFFERENT RESPONSIBILITIES	
	MENTOR	PROTÉGÉ
Clinical MS- or BS-prepared	• Provides nuts and bolts of teaching undergraduate students in clinical setting	Clinical Assistant • Pairs with seasoned MS-prepared faculty • Engages in formal or informal course on concepts of teaching and learning • Seeks feedback on a consistent basis from mentor • Stays current with evidence-based clinical nursing practices

Note: For this table, the following definitions apply: Term is a 9-month, optional renewable contract. Adjunct means employed intermittently with pay for expertise or may be considered a courtesy appointment without pay. A clinical assistant experiences the majority of employment with a partner hospital or clinic but is also employed by the university with pay to teach an undergraduate clinical section. These tables are designed to provide guidelines but are not inclusive of all responsibilities that may need to be identified by the mentor and protégé.

Major nursing organizations offer mentored leadership opportunities to learn expectations within new roles. These mentoring opportunities are invaluable but cannot replace a one-on-one mentor-protégé relationship in the workplace. Six selected programs are outlined in Table 5.4, with more detailed information available on each organization's website.

Table 5.3 provides a sample template for a PDP.

TABLE 5.3 Template for Professional Development Plan

PROFESSIONAL DEVELOPMENT PLAN (PDP) TEMPLATE

QUESTIONS	RESPONSES TO QUESTIONS	
• What are my 3- and 5-year goals? Where do I want to be in my career?		
• What do I need to accomplish to reach these goals? What are my annual objectives with measureable outcomes?		
• Whom do I need to help me be successful?		
• What are my goals and objectives for my areas of responsibility, i.e., research/scholarship, teaching/ advising, and service (college, university, and professional)?		
• Which strategies do I need to implement to reach my yearly objectives so that I am doing what I aspire to in 3 and 5 years?		
Strategy	Plan	Timeline
A.		
B. etc.		

Note: Review the list of questions in Banks (2012) and the tool template in Garand et al. (2010) for additional help in developing a PDP. Consult your university and college (department) standards document for expectations.

TABLE 5.4 Mentored Leadership Opportunities

ORGANIZATION CONTACT INFORMATION	APPLICANT	DESCRIPTION OF THE MENTORED LEADERSHIP OPPORTUNITY
American Association of Colleges of Nursing (AACN) www.aacn.nche.edu	Aspiring or new dean	Leadership for Academic Nursing • Annual selection of 55 to 60 Fellows engaged in professional development activities who aspire to become leaders in academic nursing. • Funded in part by the Helene Fuld Trust Fund. • Fellow is assessed for current leadership style and skills; has mentoring opportunities from an experienced dean; and works to accomplish identified goals.
National League for Nursing (NLN) www.nln.org		**The NLN Leadership Institute**

	Aspiring or new dean	• Annual selection of a cohort of 30.
		• Funded in part by the Johnson & Johnson Foundation.
		• Designed to:
		  • Enhance career opportunities and leadership skills
		  • Examine key issues in organizational dynamics
		  • Identify ways to develop effective high performing teams
		  • Develop the art of negotiation and communication within groups
		  • Create a 5-year, focused career plan
		  • Implement an individual plan for leadership development

ORGANIZATION CONTACT INFORMATION	APPLICANT	DESCRIPTION OF THE MENTORED LEADERSHIP OPPORTUNITY

	Experienced nurse educator who wishes to assume a leadership role in simulation	Leadership Development Program for Simulation Educators
		• Annual selection of 20 nurse educators.
		• Nurse educator is responsible for tuition and travel.
		• Designed to:
		  • Discuss the simulation initiatives of major national and international organizations
		  • Work on a group project that creates or expands simulation content for the web-based Simulation Innovation Resource Center (SIRC)
		  • Create a 3-year focused career development plan
		  • Implement an individual plan for leadership development

Robert Wood Johnson (RWJ) www.rwjfleaders.org These are four (of several) examples of RWJ leadership offerings.	Senior-level nurses Postdoctoral scholars Senior-level faculty leaders	Robert Wood Johnson Foundation Programs for Career and Leadership Development • Executive Nurse Leaders: Offers senior-level nurses a 3-year leadership program that strengthens their ability to improve America's health care system. • Health and Society Scholars: Offers 2 years of support to postdoctoral scholars in the hope of producing leaders who will improve the nation's health by addressing the full spectrum of factors that affect health and inform policy.

continues

TABLE 5.4 Continued

ORGANIZATION CONTACT INFORMATION	APPLICANT	DESCRIPTION OF THE MENTORED LEADERSHIP OPPORTUNITY
		• Health Policy Fellows: Offers exceptional mid-career health professionals and behavioral and social scientists a 1-year (or longer) residential experience in Washington, D.C., that prepares them to influence the future of health care and accelerate their own career development. • Nurse Faculty Scholars: 12 awards of up to $350,000 over 3 years to develop national leaders in academic nursing.
Sigma Theta Tau International (STTI) www.nursing society.org	Faculty member between 2 and 5 years in role	Nursing Faculty Leadership Academy (NFLA) • NFLA seeks applications from nurses who are transitioning from nursing practice to a faculty role and are committed to making nursing education a lifelong career. • Mentor is selected from a different university in the area of the faculty applicant's teaching and research area. • Commitment from faculty member's dean for institutional support. • Additional information on the website.
International Council of Nurses (ICN) www.icn.ch	Available for new leaders	Leadership for Change Program The program prepares nurses for leadership roles in nursing and the health system during reform and change. Mentoring is an essential component of this program.

ORGANIZATION CONTACT INFORMATION	APPLICANT	DESCRIPTION OF THE MENTORED LEADERSHIP OPPORTUNITY
Royal College of Nursing (RCN) www.rcn.org.uk	New members of RCN	The RCN mentors are key in preparing and supporting members for competent practice. Mentors help the members further develop their ability to reflect, learn from, and change their practice. This provides a consistent standard of care across the United Kingdom.

Role of Dean in Facilitating Mentoring

The nursing dean sets the expectations and provides resources for the process of mentoring to occur. The dean is primarily responsible for recruitment and retention of qualified faculty members. However, retention is supported by seasoned and peer faculty mentors who provide the coaching and support for novice faculty to integrate into the culture of the academic setting. Mentors are selected by the dean and department heads who are interested in providing guidance for the next generation (Erikson, 1963) and have a high level of emotional intelligence (Goleman, 1995).

The American Association of Colleges of Nursing produces an annual report on faculty vacancies to post on its website (http://www.aacn.nche.edu/news/articles/2012/enrollment-data). The 2011 report indicates that 75,587 qualified students were turned away from nursing programs because of faculty shortages. Recruitment and retention challenges for sufficient, well-prepared faculty include low salaries compared with similar education and responsibilities in service institutions; "aging-out" of current faculty; reluctance of younger nurses to pursue advanced education; tuition and loan burden for graduate education; declining enrollment in graduate studies; heavy faculty role expectations; and alternate career opportunities with a higher level of life-work balance. The dean and department heads must be aware of these factors and negotiate with the provost for competitive salaries and workload balance.

Conclusion

In the final analysis, a mentor-protégé relationship is beneficial to retention in the academic setting because of the personal satisfaction and professional success that occur. The mentor and protégé develop together, think more broadly, and learn and grow in facilitating student learning. In addition to the one-to-one relationship between the mentor and protégé, support of the process is essential from the dean and the provost. Financial support is needed for travel to conferences for professional networking, presentation of scholarship outcomes, and participation in mentored leadership opportunities described in Table 5.4. The tenure and promotion guidelines are established by the university. Performance standards are tailored for the discipline of nursing by the college and provide the framework for expected outcomes of the faculty protégé. The mentor provides the guidance to the protégé in this process at the novice, mid-career, and experienced level.

Faculty on a non-tenure track also need ongoing mentoring to meet performance expectations, engage in the work of the academic setting, and provide sustained excellence in student success. This chapter described activities and resources that facilitate the mentor-protégé process in the academic setting.

References

Advisory Board Company. (2009). *Models of faculty mentoring: Approaches at six institutions.* Washington, D.C.: Author.

Anibas, M., Brenner, G. H., & Zorn, C. R. (2009). Experiences described by novice teaching academic staff in baccalaureate nursing education: A focus on mentoring. *Journal of Professional Nursing, 25*(4), 211–217.

Banks, J. (2012). Development of scholarly trajectories that reflect core values and priorities: A strategy for promoting faculty retention. *Journal of Professional Nursing, 28*(6), 351–359.

Bland, C. J., Taylor, A. L., Shollen, S. L., Weber-Main, A. M., & Mulcahy, P. A. (2009). *Faculty success through mentoring: A guide for mentors, mentees, and leaders.* New York, NY: Rowman and Littlefield and American Council on Education (ACE).

Brendtro, M., & Hegge, M. (2000). Nursing faculty: One generation away from extinction? *Journal of Professional Nursing, 16*(2), 97– 103.

Bunkers, S. S. (2005). A community of scholars: What is it? *Nursing Science Quarterly, 18,* 117–119.

Campinha-Bacote, J. (2010). A culturally conscious model of mentoring. *Nurse Educator, 35*(3), 130–135.

Clark, N. J., Alcala-Van Houten, L., & Perea-Ryan, M. (2010). Transitioning from clinical practice to academia: University expectations on the tenure track. *Nurse Educator, 35*(3), 105–109.

Daloz, L. A. (1986). *Effective teaching and mentoring: Realizing the transformational power of adult learning experiences.* San Francisco, CA: Jossey-Bass.

Dalton, G., Thompson, P., & Price, R. (1977, Summer). The four stages of professional careers. *Organizational Dynamics, 6,* 19–42.

Dunham-Taylor, J., Lynn, C. W., Moore, P., McDaniel, S., & Walker, J. K. (2008). What goes around comes around: Improving faculty retention through more effective mentoring. *Journal of Professional Nursing, 24*(6), 337–346.

Erikson, E. (1963). *Childhood and society* (3rd ed.). New York, NY: Norton.

Garand, L., Matthews, J. T., Courtney, J. L., Davies, M., Lingler, J. H., Schlenk, E. A., . . . Burke, L. E. (2010). Development and use of a tool to guide junior faculty in their progression toward promotion and tenure. *Journal of Professional Nursing, 26*(4), 207–213.

Goleman, D. (1995). *Emotional intelligence: Why it can matter more than IQ.* New York, NY: Bantam Books.

Gwyn, P. G. (2011). The quality of mentoring relationships' impact on occupational commitment of nursing faculty. *Journal of Professional Nursing, 27*(5), 292–298.

Hegge, M., Bunkers, S., Letcher, D., Craig, G., Klawiter, R., Olson, R., . . . Winterboer, V. (2010). Clinical academic partnership: Mutual ownership for clinical learning. *Nurse Educator, 35*(2), 61–65.

Heinrich, K. T., & Oberleitner, M. G. (2012). How a faculty group's peer mentoring of each other's scholarship can enhance retention and recruitment. *Journal of Professional Nursing, 28*(1), 5–12.

Jacelon, C. S., Zucker, D. M., Staccarini, J. M., & Henneman, E. A. (2003). Peer mentoring for tenure-track faculty. *Journal of Professional Nursing, 19*(6), 335–338.

Martin, C. T., & Hodge, M. (2011). A nursing department faculty-mentored research project. *Nurse Educator, 36*(1), 35–39.

Sawatzky, J. V., & Enns, C. L. (2009). A mentoring needs assessment: Validating mentorship in nursing education. *Journal of Professional Nursing, 25*(3), 145–150.

Slimmer, L. (2012). A teaching mentorship program to facilitate excellence in teaching and learning. *Journal of Professional Nursing, 28*(3), 182–185.

Vance, C. (2011). *Fast facts for career success in nursing: Making the most of mentoring in a nutshell.* New York, NY: Springer.

Vance, C., & Olson, R. K. (1998). *The mentor connection in nursing.* New York, NY: Springer.

Zimmerman, L., & Yeaworth, R. (1985). Factors influencing career success in nursing. *Research in Nursing & Health, 9,* 179–185.

Chapter 6
Challenges of the Health Care System and the Need for Mentoring

Kristina S. Ibitayo and Susan M. Baxley

The idea that nurses "eat their young" has health care systems searching for creative ways to promote nurse creativity and initiative and ultimately to recruit and retain nurses (Latham, Hogan, & Ringl, 2008). Health care systems have used preceptor programs, and more recently mentoring programs, to assist nurses in transitioning into new roles within the organizations. The terms "preceptor" and "mentor" have sometimes been used interchangeably, with precepting being an assigned relationship for students or new nurses (Grossman, 2007; Grossman, 2013). Precepting programs use experienced nurses to help new employees transition into health care systems (Grossman, 2007; Grossman, 2013), whereas mentoring programs provide opportunities for networking and long-term career success (Benson, Morahan, Sachdeva, & Richman, 2002).

Looking at the context and time of a relationship provides a method for viewing the differences between mentoring, clinical supervision, and precepting (Mills, Francis, and Bonner, 2005). Mentoring occurs "outside the immediate work setting as it is a long-term relationship with different phases" (p. 6); clinical supervision occurs "within the work setting, but away from the immediate work area" (p. 6) and is also a long-term relationship; precepting occurs "within the work setting" (p. 6) and is a short-term relationship that typically lasts between 2 and 12 weeks. In the health care system, mentoring can influence patient outcomes and nursing staff retention. The culture of each health care organization and the systems within it influence the success of mentoring relationships.

The Culture of a Mentoring Environment

Formal mentoring programs are only successful if they are a part of the organization's culture (Colonghi, 2009), receive leadership support with designated individual(s) to staff and maintain the program, and include formal evaluation structures (Grindel & Hagerstrom, 2009). One of the first steps in initiating a mentoring program within an organization is to understand the culture of the organization as a whole as well as the individual units. Using Leininger's (1988, p. 156) definition, culture refers to the "learned, shared, and transmitted values, beliefs, norms, and life practices of a particular group that guides thinking, decisions, and actions in patterned ways." This definition helps organizations begin to define the culture that frames the life of the organizations' employees. The culture of the workplace is based on the "ethnic pride" of employees and the culture of the organization (Washington, Erickson, & Ditomassi, 2004).

Because the organization's culture provides the employees with a framework for their daily lives (Latham et al., 2008), health care organizations with positive work environments demonstrate support for increasing nursing knowledge in their organizations and implementing that knowledge in nursing practice (Beecroft, Dorey, & Wenten, 2008). A health care organization's mission, vision, and value statements are supported by mentoring relationships as employees make these values real (McKinley, 2004).

A health care organization's workforce environment can be improved after its culture is defined (Latham et al., 2008). The culture of a health care organization is formed at the organizational level, at the unit level among nursing staff, and at the individual level, with mentoring relationships influencing the culture at all levels (Latham et al., 2008). Everyone benefits from the mentoring relationship, including the organization's units and employees, as future nursing leaders are developed and supported in an environment of commitment, teamwork, and retention (McKinley, 2004).

Health care systems today are becoming increasingly specialized and might be considered complex adaptive systems as noted by Burns in chapter 2 , who states that these systems need to allow new entities to emerge for delivery of accountable care. Burns also suggests that any change in one part of the system affects other parts as well.

Today's work environment often includes constantly changing demands, so conflict arises if there are scheduling constraints between mentoring functions and job duties (Beecroft, Santner, Lacy, Kunzman, & Dorey, 2006). However, a commitment to the mentoring relationship is even more important to its success than is the actual time allotted for the mentor and protégé to meet (Beecroft et al., 2006). In addition to an organization's provision of role training and allotment of time for mentoring, mentors and protégés need to commit to meeting regularly so that their mentoring connection can grow and be successful (Beecroft et al., 2006). Mentoring programs that include formalized training for mentors and protégés increase the effectiveness of the mentoring relationship from 30 percent to 90 percent (Dancer, 2003).

Mentors are typically older, wiser, more experienced, and have more authority than their protégés (Beecroft et al., 2006). Mentoring should be voluntary rather than required (Colonghi, 2009). Not everyone can be a mentor, as a mentor must draw on abilities and experiences with "a high degree of motivation and commitment to the profession, the organization, and the growth of the mentee" (McKinley, 2004, p. 209). Ideal mentors are positive individuals who build trust, are self-aware, and demonstrate commitment to their own professional development; however, certain individuals, such as "the fixer, the bureaucrat, the pleaser, and the talker" (Tabbron, Macaulay, & Cook, 1997, p. 8), are ineffective mentors. In the initial phases of the mentoring relationship, the mentor may be more proactive in contacting the protégé (Mcdonald, Mohan, Jackson, Vickers, & Wilkes, 2010), but with the help of the mentor, the protégé must be the driving force in deciding which outcomes are desired (Dancer, 2003).

Nurses Seeking New Positions After Graduation

Graduates from nursing programs face varied challenges. There are similarities and differences, depending on the level of nursing experience prior to graduation and the degree level obtained. Mentoring strategies employed in the health care setting have been shown to increase nurse productivity, enhance leadership skills and organizational communication, increase job satisfaction, and promote nurse retention (Gordon & Melrose, 2011). But despite a mentoring strategy employed by a health care system, some nurses who have specific career plans may not experience increased job satisfaction or commit long-term to an organization (Raabe & Beehr, 2003; Willits, 2009). Mentoring relationships that are successful in the health care system include a strong socialization aspect, where mentors and protégés may meet outside the organization, and where protégés may select their own mentors (Persaud, 2008). One of the major difficulties protégés experience is finding time to communicate with their mentors and establish regular meetings (Willits, 2009). Health care organizations that have successful mentoring programs need to establish a supportive mentoring culture and ensure that time is allotted for the development of these relationships.

A mentor's professionalism and attitude in the work setting assist a protégé's adaptation to the workplace, provide an example to emulate, and enhance a protégé's commitment and loyalty to the organization (Weng et al., 2010). An organization that commits to the success of its mentoring program invests in the development of its nurse leaders (Colonghi, 2009). In turn, the attitude of nurse leaders and the value placed on nursing staff positively influence the job satisfaction of nurses in that health care organization (Colonghi, 2009). In a Taiwan study, job satisfaction for new nurses was highest when role-modeling was used, and, due to the trust and respect inherent in the mentoring relationship, the protégés attempted to imitate the mentors to improve their nursing skills (Weng et al., 2010).

Successful mentoring programs based in an organizational environment that supports professional nursing practice and shared governance ease the transition for new graduates into the health care system (Halfer, Graf, & Sullivan, 2008). A mentor nurtures the new nurse by having an attitude open to discussion and assisting the protégé in understanding the work environment's social culture (Persaud, 2008). In contrast, nurse leaders profit from mentors by learning the skill set of determination, the ability to navigate in a complex environment, and the necessity of seeking advice and support as needed (Colonghi, 2009).

TIPS on Mentoring New Nurses

To minimize bachelor of science in nursing (BSN) graduates' anxiety and stress in their first nursing jobs, it is important that they experience a supportive environment (Beecroft et al., 2008). Individual nurses can utilize five strategies to decrease professional isolation and gain encouragement in their professional practice: sharing their stories with peers, reflecting on past experiences, recalling prior role models, adopting an attitude of continuous learning, and mentoring students (Gordon & Melrose, 2011). New nurses also benefit from mentors' guidance as they learn organizational values (Dancer, 2003). In addition, good mentors guide protégés by helping them focus on "challenges, choices, consequences, creative solutions, and conclusions" (Pegg, 1999, p. 136). Health care systems with caring environments invest in the mentoring process to develop the performance of their skilled workforce (Dancer, 2003). Effective mentors have credibility, show warmth toward their protégés, and are "sage-like and street-wise" (Pegg, 1999, p. 136).

TIPS on Mentoring Nurses in New Roles

As nurse practitioner (NP) students transition into their role as new NPs in primary care practices, they benefit from mentoring relationships in the areas of "quality of care, productivity, job satisfaction, and longevity" (Harrington, 2011, p. 171). These same benefits could apply to all nurses in a new role. When experienced NPs take on the role of mentoring new NPs, they need to consider whether they have the qualifications and skills needed to be effective. Several aspects should be considered, including (Hayes & Gagan, 2005, p. 443):

- Maturity

- Strong interpersonal skills

- Clinical, teaching, administrative, and research skills

- Organizational political knowledge and skills

- Competence and confidence in the role of NP

- Commitment, loyalty, and leadership to the organization

- Access to organizational resources

- Knowledge of the workings of the organizational environment

NPs' experiences with mentors may heavily influence whether the protégés become valuable health care providers who make significant contributions to the outcomes of their patients (Hayes, 1998). When NPs' mentors use the Tao approach to mentoring, there is an "emphasis on empathy, compassion, nurturing, mutual respect, and learning" (Hayes, 1998, p. 57), resulting in the protégés' socialization into the system and their commitment to patients. The Tao approach to mentoring "is a two-way circular dance that provides opportunities to experience both giving and receiving without limitations and fears" (Huang & Lynch, 1995, p. xii).

Mentorship has a significant impact on a nurse executive's career mobility and influence in the nursing organization (Moran, Duffield, Donoghue, Stasa, & Blay, 2011). To be effective in mentoring minority protégés, mentors need these five competencies: "candor, compromise, confidence, complexity, and champion" (Washington et al., 2004, p. 168). Mentors for junior nurse executives are typically experienced nurse executives who serve as mentors primarily for personal satisfaction, because they have been mentored, and because they now want to assist the next generation (Finley, Ivanitskaya, & Kennedy, 2007).

TRANSITION TO A NURSE RESEARCHER IN A HEALTH CARE SYSTEM

As health care organizations seek and maintain Magnet Recognition status desiring to provide quality patient care and nursing excellence, they recognize the need for nurse researchers. During an interview about her new role as a nurse researcher, Marygrace Hernandez-Leveille, PhD, RN, ACNP-BC, shared her thoughts on mentoring from the perspective of a protégé and a mentor. As Hernandez-Leveille was mentored into her new role as a nurse researcher, her mentors had the attributes of "openness and a willingness to share their knowledge and experience" (M. Hernandez-Leveille, personal communication, February 5, 2013). Everyone was open to reiterating new things so that she could ultimately be successful: "That was the organization's goal, for me to be successful and not experience a setup for failure" (M. Hernandez-Leveille, personal communication, February 5, 2013). The mentoring process was primarily informal, done in person or via emails and phone calls.

Hernandez-Leveille believes precepting means orienting someone to a new role similar to that of the preceptor, as when she precepted other NPs in their new NP roles. According to Hernandez-Leveille, "There is a difference in mentoring, as I now mentor nurses in the research process and make myself available to the nurses, accommodating their schedule, visiting with them personally, emailing and calling them, and orienting them to the librarian so that they learn how to perform literature searches" (personal communication, February 5, 2013).

Hernandez-Leveille offers the following tips for protégés in a beginning research role:

- *Always be positive.*

- *Do not take no for an answer—figure out how you can accomplish your goal.*

- *Have perseverance and tenacity.*

- *Pick a research topic you have a passion for and are interested in so that you can stay engaged.*

TIPS on Mentoring International Nurses

In this chapter, the term *international nurses* refers to nurses who are born outside the United States but may have received their education in their home countries and/or in the United States. International nurses face the challenge of understanding a nursing culture that may be radically different than what they have experienced or had knowledge of in their home countries (Ibitayo, 2010). Not only do international nurses experience different nursing cultures within the health facilities where they are employed, but they are also expected to understand and navigate within a societal culture that may differ from their own (Ibitayo, 2010). They may need help communicating effectively with patients, their families, and other health team members (Ryan, 2010). After hire, international nurses may benefit from transition programs provided by their employers to assist them in adapting to their new practice environment (Zizzo & Xu, 2009). In the United Kingdom, when international nurses, mentors, and employees expectations differed in the transition program, those expectations affect the quality of supervision (Xu & He, 2012). When English is a second language, international nurses face the added challenge of understanding the nuances of communication particular to American society at large. Transition programs are needed because of required language proficiency, and when comparing the U.S. to the international nurse's country of origin, there are differences in "nursing education, national health care systems, nursing practice, and culture" (Xu & He, 2012, p. 223). Some things that help internationally educated nurses (IENs) transition to the U.S. health care system include having experienced mentors who are also international nurses, presenting the experiences of IENs to American nurses, and participating in comprehensive orientation programs (Ryan, 2010). Another mentoring option is cross-cultural mentoring, which "occurs between two individuals that differ in at least two of the following cultural categories: race, class, gender" (Blanchett & Clarke-Yapi, 1999, p. 49).

Mentoring Programs in a Health Care System

Successful mentoring programs should include these key factors: "a clear agreed set of objectives, communications and training, matching of mentors and mentees, [and] evaluation and review of programme" (Tabbron et al., 1997, p. 8). Generational differences in learning as well as individual learning styles should be considered when implementing mentoring programs (Latham et al., 2008). Johnson (2002, p. 91) suggests that participants in programs consider the structure of the mentoring relationship, provide consent for the mentoring assignment, avoid sexual intimacies between mentors and protégés, and consider when it is appropriate to interrupt or terminate the relationship to ensure the maintenance of ethical principles. Some of the failures in mentoring programs occur when expectations for the relationship are unrealistic, the mentor does not have time allotted for meeting with the protégé, generational and social differences between the protégé and the mentor are not understood, and appropriate funding is lacking (Martindale, McClave, Heylend, & August, 2010).

Hayes and Scott (2007) report on a program in which a health care facility collaborated with a university to provide faculty for mentoring new nurses. A faculty member taught a course that consisted of one-on-one support for new graduates during their first few weeks of employment. The faculty member was paid by the health care facility, and the course provided access to the faculty member as well as weekly seminars. The faculty provided coaching and support to assist the new graduates to gain confidence in their new roles. The program showed success over the first 2 years it was in existence, with a 100% retention rate of the new nurses.

This program is similar to a program initiated by Susan Baxley to provide extensive hands-on learning for new nurses in a labor and delivery area. Baxley provided the nurses with support, coaching, ways to navigate the personalities of the seasoned nurses and physicians, and tips for the promotion of their long-term goals. This program was successful in retaining nurses but also in providing the participants with the skills to make future decisions about the career paths they wanted to pursue. One of the key purposes of mentors in the health care clinical setting is to ensure that protégés experience a nurturing environment with appropriate learning opportunities and resources (Gopee, 2007).

Planning for compatibility of mentors and protégés may assist in promoting the relationships within the parameters of the ethical principles (Harrington, 2011). Although ideal mentors may be matched using compatibility tests and interest assessments, mentors can also be assigned to protégés without testing procedures, and these mentoring relationships may flourish because of the unique talents and knowledge both mentor and protégé possess (Beecroft et al., 2006). Mentors may also be matched with protégés who have different strengths than theirs (Beecroft et al., 2006), but proximity, access, availability to travel, personal and professional interests, and gender should also be considered (McDonald et al., 2010).

Conclusion

Health care systems struggle to provide leadership as they are in a state of change, necessitating thinking outside established parameters and providing different solutions than those the organizations have traditionally implemented. Some of these changes relate to how the organization provides orientation and support to nurses in new roles and how they are integrated into the organization's culture and the profession of nursing. Within a health care organization, the mentoring process provides stakeholders with the skills and motivation to achieve personal goals and to help develop the ideal organization they envision (Dancer, 2003). This culture of mentoring provides an advantage to health care systems as they provide support for employees. A mentoring relationship's outcomes are broad, resulting in "improved clinical practice, career progression, scholarly endeavour, [and] personal achievement" (Mills et al., 2005, p. 6). An organization's mentoring culture also benefits nurses who have emigrated from other countries. After relocating from their home countries, these nurses may face multiple barriers, such as language fluency in communication, different clinical practices, immigration challenges, and verification of qualifications (Kingma, 2006).

No statistically significant measurable outcomes verify the influence of mentoring programs on career satisfaction and intent to stay in nursing, because nurses may stay in the profession for a variety of reasons, such as job security, the altruistic value of nursing, the caring aspect of nursing, and lack of other career options (Mariani, 2007). Additional research is needed among younger generations of nurses to determine whether mentoring programs influence their career satisfaction (Mariani, 2007). Leaders in all levels of health care organizations need to reinforce the value of generational differences in their employees by considering the positive contributions of generational mentoring when forming teams and establishing mentoring relationships (Stewart, 2006).

In summary, "[a] mentor points to doors—they don't open them. But they enable you to find the strength to open them yourself " (Standing Committee on Post Dental and Medical Education, 1998, p. 1).

References

Beecroft, P. C., Dorey, F., & Wenten, M. (2008). Turnover intention in new graduate nurses: A multivariate analysis. *Journal of Advanced Nursing, 62*(1), 41–52. doi:10.1111/j.1365-648.2007.04570.x

Beecroft, P. C., Santner, S., Lacy, M. L., Kunzman, L., & Dorey, F. (2006). New graduate nurses' perceptions of mentoring: Six-year programme evaluation. *Journal of Advanced Nursing, 55*(6), 736–747. doi:10.1111/j.1365-2648.2006.03964.x

Benson, C. A., Morahan, P. S., Sachdeva, A. K., & Richman, R. C. (2002). Effective faculty preceptoring and mentoring during reorganization of an academic medical center. *Medical Teacher, 24*(5), 550–557. doi:10.1080/0142159021000002612

Blanchett, W. J., & Clarke-Yapi, M. D. (1999). Cross-cultural mentoring of ethnic minority students: Implications for increasing minority faculty. *Professional Educator, 22*(1), 49–62.

Colonghi, P. (2009). Mentoring? Take the LEAD. *Nursing Management, 40*, 15–17. Retrieved from http://journals.lww.com/nursingmanagement/Pages/default.aspx

Dancer, J. M. (2003). Mentoring in healthcare: Theory in search of practice? *Clinician in Management, 12*(1), 21–31. Retrieved from http://www.ingentaconnect.com/content/rmp/cim

Finley, F. R., Ivanitskaya, L. V., & Kennedy, M. H. (2007). Mentoring junior healthcare administrators: A description of mentoring practices in 127 U.S. hospitals . . . including commentary by Hofmann PB. *Journal of Healthcare Management, 52*(4), 260–270. http://www.ache.org/Publications/SubscriptionPurchase. aspx#jhm

Gopee, N. (2007). *Mentoring and Supervision in Healthcare.* London, England: SAGE.

Gordon, K. P., & Melrose, S. (2011). Self-mentoring: Five practical strategies to improve retention of long-term care staff. *Canadian Nursing Home, 22*(2), 14–19. Retrieved from http://www. nursinghomemagazine.ca/index.html

Grindel, C. G., & Hagerstrom, G. (2009). Nurses nurturing nurses: Outcomes and lessons learned. *MEDSURG Nursing, 18*(3), 183–187. Retrieved from http://www.medsurgnursing.net/cgi-bin/ WebObjects/MSNJournal.woa

Grossman, S. C. (2007). *Mentoring in nursing: A dynamic and collaborative process.* New York, NY: Springer.

Grossman, S. C. (2013). *Mentoring in nursing: A dynamic and collaborative process* (2nd ed.). New York, NY: Springer.

Halfer, D., Graf, E., & Sullivan, C. (2008). The organizational impact of a new graduate pediatric nurse mentoring program. *Nursing Economic$, 26*(4), 243–249. Retrieved from http://www. nursingeconomics.net/cgi-bin/WebObjects/NECJournal.woa

Harrington, S. (2011). Mentoring new nurse practitioners to accelerate their development as primary care providers: A literature review. *Journal of the American Academy of Nurse Practitioners, 23*(4), 168–174. doi:10.1111/j.1745-7599.2011.00601.x

Hayes, E. (1998). Mentoring and self-efficacy for advanced nursing practice: A philosophical approach for nurse practitioner preceptors. *Journal of the American Academy of Nurse Practitioners, 10*(2), 53–57. doi:10.1111/j.1745-7599.1998. tb00495.x

Hayes, E. F. & Gagan, M. J. (2005). Fellows column. Approaches to mentoring: How to mentor and be mentored. *Journal of the American Academy of Nurse Practitioners, 17*(11), 442–445. doi:10.1111/j.1745-7599.2005.0008.x

Hayes, J. M., & Scott, A. S. (2007). Mentoring partnerships as the wave of the future for new graduates. *Nursing Education Perspectives, 28*(1), 27–29. Retrieved from http://www.nlnjournal.org/Doi/pdf/10.1043/1536-5026%282007%29028%5B0027%3AMPATWO%5D2.0.CO% 3B2

Huang, C. A. & Lynch, J. (1995). *Mentoring: The Tao of giving and receiving wisdom.* San Francisco, CA: Harper.

Ibitayo, K. S. (2010). *Factors affecting the relocation and transition of internationally educated nurses migrating to the United States of America.* (Doctoral dissertation). Retrieved from ProQuest Dissertations and Theses database. (UMI No. 3439696)

Johnson, W. B. (2002). The intentional mentor: Strategies and guidelines for the practice of mentoring. *Professional Psychology: Research and Practice, 33*(1), 88–96. doi:10.1037/0735-7028.33.1.88

Kingma, M. (2006). *Nurses on the Move: Migration and the Global Health Care Economy.* Ithaca, NY: Cornell University Press.

Latham, C. L., Hogan, M., & Ringl, K. (2008). Nurses supporting nurses: Creating a mentoring program for staff nurses to improve the workforce environment. *Nursing Administration Quarterly, 32*(1), 27–39. doi:10.1097/01.naq.0000305945.23569.2b

Leininger, M. (1988). Leininger's theory of nursing: Cultural care diversity and universality. *Nursing Science Quarterly, 1*(4), 152–160. Retrieved from http://nsq.sagepub.com/content/1/4.toc

Mariani, B. S. (2007). *The effect of mentoring on career satisfaction of registered nurses and intent to stay in the nursing profession* (Doctoral dissertation). Retrieved from ProQuest Dissertations and Theses database. (UMI No. 3272377)

Martindale, R. G., McClave, S., Heyland, D., & August, D. (2010). Developing a mentoring program in clinical nutrition. *Journal of Parenteral and Enteral Nutrition, 34*(Supplement 1): 70S-77S. doi:10.1177/0148607110376199

McDonald, G., Mohan, S., Jackson, D., Vickers, M. H., & Wilkes, L. (2010). Continuing connections: The experiences of retired and senior working nurse mentors. *Journal of Clinical Nursing, 19*(23), 3547–3554. doi:10.1111/j.1365-2702.2010.03365.x

McKinley, M. G. (2004). Mentoring matters: Creating, connecting, empowering. *AACN Clinical Issues: Advanced Practice in Acute and Critical Care, 15*(2), 205–214. doi:10.1097/00044067-200404000-00005

Mills, J. E., Francis, K. L., & Bonner, A. (2005). Mentoring, clinical supervision and preceptoring: Clarifying the conceptual definitions for Australian rural nurses. A review of the literature. *Rural and Remote Health, 5*(3), 1–10. Retrieved from http://www.rrh.org.au/publishedarticles/article_print_410.pdf

Moran, P., Duffield, C. M., Donoghue, J., Stasa, H., & Blay, N. (2011). Factors impacting on career progression for nurse executives. *Contemporary Nurse, 38*(1–2), 45–55. doi:10.5172/conu.2011.38.1-2.45

Pegg, M. (1999). The art of mentoring. *Industrial and Commercial Training, 31*(4), 136. doi:10.1108/00197859910275683

Persaud, D. (2008). Mentoring the new graduate perioperative nurse: A valuable retention strategy. *AORN Journal, 87*(6), 1173. doi:10.1016/j.aorn.2007.10.014

Raabe, B., & Beehr, T. A. (2003). Formal mentoring, versus supervisor and coworker relationships: Differences in perceptions and impact. *Journal of Organizational Behavior, 24*(3), 271–293. doi:10.1002/job.193

Ryan, J. G. (2010). *Adjusting to the United States healthcare workplace: Perceptions of internationally born and educated registered nurses* (Doctoral dissertation). Retrieved from ProQuest Dissertations and Theses database. (UMI No. 3407358)

Standing Committee on Post Dental and Medical Education. (1998). *Supporting doctors and dentists at work: An inquiry into mentoring.* London, England: SCOPME.

Stewart, D. W. (2006). Generational mentoring. *Journal of Continuing Education in Nursing, 37*(3), 113–120. Retrieved from http://www.healio.com/journals/JCEN/%7B28366671-590A-4EE2-B6A5-8CC5F9B202E4%7D/Generational-Mentoring

Tabbron, A., Macaulay, S., & Cook, S. (1997). Making mentoring work. *Training for Quality, 5*(1), 6–9. doi:10.1108/09684879710156469

Washington, D., Erickson, J. I., & Ditomassi, M. (2004). Mentoring the minority nurse leader of tomorrow. *Nursing Administration Quarterly, 28*(3), 165–169. doi:10.1097/00006216-200407000-00003

Weng, R. H., Huang, C. Y., Tsai, W. C., Chang, L. Y., Lin, S. E., & Lee, M. Y. (2010). Exploring the impact of mentoring functions on job satisfaction and organizational commitment of new staff nurses. *BMC Health Services Research, 10*, 240–240. doi:10.1186/1472-6963-10-240

Willits, E. M. (2009). *Can we get nurses to stay? A qualitative study to evaluate the effectiveness of a formal mentoring program in an acute care health system* (Doctoral dissertation). Retrieved from ProQuest Dissertations and Theses database. (UMI No. 3392165).

Xu, Y., & He, F. (2012). Transition programs for internationally educated nurses: What can the United States learn from the United Kingdom, Australia, and Canada? *Nursing Economic$, 30*(4), 215–224. Retrieved from http://www.nursingeconomics.net/cgi-bin/WebObjects/NECJournal.woa

Zizzo, K. A., & Xu, Y. (2009). Post-hire transitional programs for international nurses: A systematic review. *Journal of continuing education in nursing, 40*(2), 57–66. doi: 10.3928/00220124-20090201-02

Chapter 7
Mentoring Traditions Throughout the World

Jennifer Gray, Manuel Moreno, and Esther Gallegos

Mentoring occurs in a context that shapes the purpose, tone, and structure of the mentoring relationship (Patel et al., 2011). The sociopolitical culture of the context is a significant factor in determining the norms of a mentoring relationship and the expectations the mentor and protégé bring to the relationship. This chapter contains descriptions of mentoring that were contributed by approximately 50 nursing colleagues from around the world, the majority of whom reside in Spain and Mexico. These colleagues responded to the authors' questions from their own perspectives. It is important to note that the views of these colleagues are not necessarily representative of other nurses in the same countries.

During the process of reviewing the literature and collecting information from nurses in different countries, it became evident that the concept of mentoring varies across cultures. Following a description of selected perspectives of mentoring as a concept, the impact of these variations on the roles of mentors and protégés is described. The chapter also includes exemplars of the values and traditions of mentors related to culture, gender, and religion. To conclude the chapter, factors to consider when mentoring across international boundaries and cultures are summarized.

Concept of Mentoring

Authors on mentoring frequently describe the process as being formal and informal in nature (McCloughen, O'Brien, & Jackson, 2009; Patel et al., 2011). Different modalities of mentoring emerged in conversations with colleagues from Spain and Mexico as well as other countries. Nurses in Spain identified one modality to be the tutoring a professor may give a student or the supervision an experienced nurse may provide a student (M. Moreno, personal communication, February 4, 2013). Supportive relationships that occur between nurses with less experience and nurses with more experience reflect the second type of mentoring. In Mexico, an early modality of mentoring occurred between advanced nursing students and freshmen students, who were assigned *madrinas*, or godmothers (E. Gallegos, personal communication, February 14, 2013). The madrinas were responsible for guiding new students through the adjustment to the university and the nursing program. This mentoring style disappeared and was replaced by the current modality of institutional programs in which faculty members are named as mentors for 5 to 10 students. These faculty mentors are expected to orient, accompany, and support their student mentees with the goal of degree completion.

Mentoring programs have been viewed as one way to reduce nurse turnover and promote professional satisfaction of nurses. In Vietnam and Hong Kong, new graduates are provided a formal mentor (preceptor) during their first employment (N. Hue, personal communication, January 14, 2013; A. Lai, personal communication, January 27, 2013). In Finland and Britain, Jokelainen, Jammokeeah, Tossavainen, and Turunen (2011) conducted a phenomenological study of mentoring of nursing students in organizational contexts that was based on the assumption that mentoring is dependent on an organization's capacity for supporting mentoring. In Uganda, mentoring has been shaped more by professional norms and is described as being task-oriented and an expectation in education and service settings (C. Aliga, personal communication, December 4, 2012). Even without formal mentoring per se, student nurses and recently graduated nurses are expected to take instruction and guidance from more experienced nurses in the hospital or clinic. This is similar to what was reported to occur in Hong Kong (A. Lai, personal communication, January 27, 2013). In addition to the formal mentoring programs in Hong Kong, informal mentoring occurs through interpersonal relationships between novices and nurses who are more experienced.

Formal mentoring may transition into informal mentoring over the course of a relationship. For example, mentoring was formally implemented during a U.S.-Romanian partnership in palliative care nursing but evolved from a one-way relationship into a mutually beneficial, reciprocal relationship (Vosit-Steller, Morse, & Mitrea, 2011). At the core of the mentoring relationship was collaboration based on understanding each participant's needs. When the mentoring relationship becomes reciprocal, it more closely resembles a synergistic relationship that energizes the two individuals involved, as described by a nurse in Canada (D. Martin, personal communication, December 5, 2012).

Clearly, variations exist in the concept of mentoring. As a result, when mentoring is sought across cultures, an early conversation is needed between the mentor and protégé to clarify what each believes mentoring should involve. Table 7.1 provides a summary of the types of mentoring with indicators of countries in which participants described mentoring that way. Even when a country is not identified in the table as having a specific type of mentoring, that type of mentoring may exist in the country but was not mentioned by the person interviewed or the literature reviewed.

Roles of Mentors and Mentees

The Statuary Authority in Hong Kong designates the mentor for each new graduate who is hired in the hospital. During the 2-year mentorship, the mentor is expected to support the new registered nurse (RN) in meeting professional competencies, including developing an agreement about what the protégé needs to learn to achieve the competencies (A. Lai, personal communication, January 27, 2013).

TABLE 7.1 How Mentoring Is Implemented and Experienced in Different Countries

DESCRIPTION	AUSTRALIA	CANADA	EUROPEAN COUNTRIES*	HONG KONG	MEXICO	SPAIN	UGANDA	VIETNAM
Structured linking of more advanced student with student early in the educational program (Academic support)						x		
Faculty or clinical instructor with an individual or small group of students (Academic support and supervision)	x			x	x	x		
Formal mentoring program between experienced nurses and nurses recently hired (Transition to practice)	x		x	x			x	x
Informal relationship between experienced nurses and new nurse						x		
Experienced nurse leader with less experienced leader in nonwork and nonacademic settings		x	x	x	x		x	x

Extracted from published reports of projects in Great Britain, Finland, and Romania.

A common perception across countries was that a mentor is expected to monitor the protégé's progress, including identifying strengths and weaknesses and providing opportunities to improve in areas of lower competence (Table 7.2). Patel et al. (2011, p. 421), writing about mentoring in Australia, described giving feedback as "holding up a mirror." A colleague in Uganda indicated that the mentor makes a plan to support and develop the protégé in areas of weaknesses and build on strengths (C. Aliga, personal communication, December 4, 2012). The roles shift when mentoring occurs among peers, because the purpose is different. The main goal of mentoring among peers is to create an organizational environment that simplifies teamwork, the consolidation of projects, and the achievement of academic and personal goals.

TABLE 7.2 Roles of Mentors

ROLES OF MENTORS	AUSTRALIA	CANADA	EUROPEAN COUNTRIES*	HONG KONG	MEXICO	SPAIN	UGANDA	VIETNAM
Provider of information		x	x					x
Evaluator (monitor progress, identify strengths and weaknesses)	x	x	x	x	x	x	x	x
Goal setter				x				
Provider of opportunities	x			x				
Coach and encourager	x		x	x	x			
Role model	x	x	x			x		x
Assigner of tasks						x		
Companion							x	
Promoter of teamwork					x			

Extracted from published reports of projects in Great Britain, Finland, and Romania.

TABLE 7.3 Roles of Protégés

ROLES OF PROTÉGÉS	AUSTRALIA	CANADA	EUROPEAN COUNTRIES*	HONG KONG	MEXICO	SPAIN	UGANDA	VIETNAM
Accepting of feedback				x	x	x		
Completer of assigned tasks		x				x		
Student who is willing to learn and is responsible for own learning	x	x	x	x	x	x	x	x
Apprentice	x				x		x	
Open to growth		x						
Prepared at meetings	x							

Extracted from published reports of projects in Great Britain, Finland, and Romania.

Protégés are expected to accept feedback from their mentors and to complete the tasks assigned by the mentors to the best of their abilities (Z. Black, personal communication, December 11, 2012). The common theme across colleagues was that protégés are students, in reality or in perspective, and they must be willing to learn and accept responsibility for their own learning (Table 7.3).

Protégés who are mentored may develop to the point that they become willing to mentor others. One of the expectations of the International Council of Nurses' Leadership for Change program is that participants in the program will initially be protégés but eventually assume the roles of mentors because of the training incorporated into the program (Anazor, 2012). This is a valuable goal, especially in cultures where mentoring is a professional expectation.

Cultural Values and Traditions

Cultural values and traditions (Table 7.4) are critical factors to consider when beginning a mentoring relationship. Altruism was identified as a cultural value in Mexico that promoted the desire to mentor others and sustained the relationship (E. Gallegos, personal communication, February 14, 2013).

TABLE 7.4 Cultural Values Influencing Mentoring Relationships

CULTURAL VALUES	AUSTRALIA	CANADA	EUROPEAN COUNTRIES*	HONG KONG	MEXICO	SPAIN	UGANDA	VIETNAM
Altruism					x			
Equality		x						
Paternalism					x	x		x
Mutual respect	x							
Respect for the importance of family					x	x		
Respect for age				x				
Respect for individuals and other cultures	x	x				x		
Respect for learning and advanced education							x	x
Respect for practice experience					x		x	

Extracted from published reports of projects in Great Britain, Finland, and Romania.

McCloughen et al. (2009, p. 329) echoed the importance of altruism and identified a theme of "considering each other with positive regard" in their phenomenological study of mentoring in Australia. A Ugandan participant did not mention altruism specifically but alluded to it when describing mentoring as an expectation of members of the nursing profession. Nurses in Uganda become mentors as they gain experience in the field (Z. Black, personal communication, December 11, 2012). The very experiences that give mentors the background and knowledge to share with less experienced nurses can also contribute to a power differential and attitude of paternalism between mentor and protégé. Identifying paternalism as problematic, three participants indicated that it still existed in their countries but was changing as the culture changed. Although often motivated by altruism and maintained by cultural and political systems (Kim, 2011), paternalism can have negative effects when the protégé is not allowed to make decisions independently. Supportive mentors allow protégés to make their own decisions, even when the protégé's decision differs from what the mentor would recommend (Patel et al. 2011).

Cultural change has not diminished the value of respect. Repeating what McCloughen et al. (2009) found, different types of respect were identified by participants from several countries and included mutual respect that resulted in appreciating individuals for their unique characteristics and cultural heritage. Crutcher (2007) noted that mentors who mentor people of different backgrounds must be nonjudgmental and possess awareness of their own cultural values and biases.

Gender Roles

The cultural value of respect can be linked to the effects of gender on the mentoring relationship. Gender roles were the area of greatest contrast across countries. Participants indicated that, in some countries and settings, gender had little or no effect on mentoring (Table 7.5). The limited effect of gender may be due to few male nurses in some countries, resulting in few male-female mentoring relationships. Power differences between the genders were still evident in the descriptions of several participants. Women were described as being viewed as caregivers, dependent on men, and lacking confidence. Men, in contrast, were viewed as being more oriented toward technology and seeing themselves as being experts.

TABLE 7.5 Gender Roles' Influence on Mentoring Relationships

GENDER ROLES	AUSTRALIA	CANADA	EUROPEAN COUNTRIES*	HONG KONG	MEXICO	SPAIN	UGANDA	VIETNAM
Gender has little or no effect on mentoring.					x	x		
Same-gender mentoring is the norm.		x			x		x	x
Women are viewed as more dependent or lacking confidence.	x				x		x	
Women are caregivers.						x		
Men are technically focused.	x					x		

Extracted from published reports of projects in Great Britain, Finland, and Romania.

Colleagues in Spain and Australia indicated that cultural values and gender roles were evolving due to globalization and migration of nurses and other professionals in health care. One response to the increase in migration of health care professionals has been the initiation of the European Directive 36 to harmonize professional standards (Nichols, Davis, & Richardson, 2011). The European Directive 36 was disseminated to facilitate movement of professionals across national borders because their professional competencies and regulations would be consistent (European Commission, 2011). This initiative may harmonize standards but will not negate the need for mentors who are aware of potential differences in cultural, gender, and religious values across countries.

Religious Values and Practices

Although gender roles differed by location, the effects of religious values and practices on mentoring were similar across countries. The repeated theme was that the organization and setting determined the influence of religious values on mentoring. In religiously affiliated hospitals and universities, religious values and practices were powerful influences on the relationships between mentors and protégés. Colleagues in Spain explained this as the influence of the Catholic faith on mentoring in Catholic-supported institutions (M. Moreno, personal communication, February 4, 2013). In secular organizations across Spain and other countries, however, not only did religion not affect mentoring, but there was some degree of recoil away from religion.

Barriers to Mentoring

Some conversations with colleagues about mentoring included references to barriers. Colleagues in Vietnam, Mexico, and Australia stated that a lack of time was a significant barrier to mentoring (N. Hue, personal communication, January 14, 2013; E. Gallegos, personal communication, February 14, 2013; R. Rossiter, personal communication, January 11, 2013). A nurse from Hong Kong described the busy clinical environment as a barrier, because mentoring was not part of the nurse's job description and, thus, not built into the daily routines of the nurse (A. Lai, personal communication, January 14, 2013). Personalities of mentors and protégés and attitudes of managers were described by others as being barriers to effective mentoring. Another frequently mentioned barrier was the lack of mentor training. Training can prepare the mentor to maintain a dual perspective of acknowledging the protégé's individualism and group or societal membership (Crutcher, 2007).

Conclusion

When a mentor and a protégé are from different countries or ethnic groups within the same country, establishing a relationship requires openness to differences and mutual respect for each other's beliefs. As suggested by these colleagues, differences exist across organizations as well as countries and cultures (see also Chapter 2), and they can enrich or derail a mentoring relationship. Effective, supportive relationships do not occur by accident and may require training for mentors. Mentors may benefit from learning about potential differences across countries, while recognizing that each person is more than the individual's racial or ethnic heritage. As each new generation of nurses enters the profession, and less experienced nurses seek guidance from more experienced leaders, mentoring is the human connection that can bridge and transcend differences across backgrounds and individuals.

NURSES WHO PROVIDED INFORMATION FOR THE CHAPTER

Cliff Asher Aliga is the Coordinator, Uganda Wellness Centre for Health Care Workers, Kampala, Uganda. Aliga was a staff nurse and nursing officer at International Hospital Kampala and Fort Portal Regional Referral Hospital prior to becoming the Coordinator of the Wellness Centre. The Wellness Centre was opened in 2011 with support from the Ugandan government and international partners and donors (Carrier-Walker, 2011). The purpose of the Wellness Centre is to provide treatment and prevention services for nurses and other health care workers, especially those living with HIV/AIDS infection.

Zakayo Masereka Black is the Executive Secretary of the Uganda Nurses and Midwives Union (UNMU). Black persevered through numerous challenges and earned his baccalaureate in nursing science when he was 44 years old from the Ugandan Christian University. The UNMU is the professional nursing organization in Uganda and is a member of the International Council of Nurses.

Esther Gallegos (co-author) obtained input from six colleagues, three in Mexico and three in South America, who chose to remain unidentified.

Nguyen Thi Hue, BA, is a lecturer at Nam Dinh University of Nursing, Nam Dinh City, Vietnam. Nam Dinh University of Nursing is a multidisciplinary university that is over 50 years old.

Adela Lai, MHA, MBA, FHKAN, FHKCHSE, is a Professional Consultant for The Nethersole School of Nursing and a member of the Faculty of Medicine, The Chinese University of Hong Kong. She spent her career as a nurse in an acute care hospital. Since her retirement, she has been developing a leadership development program at the School of Nursing.

continues

continued

Dianne Martin, RPN, RN, BScN, MA, is the Executive Director of the Registered Practical Nurses Association of Ontario (RPNAO), Canada. She spent 26 years as a bedside nurse before becoming a senior policy analyst for the Ministry of Health and Long Term Care in Ontario.

Manuel Moreno, co-author, obtained input from 22 colleagues in Spain who chose to remain unidentified.

Rachel Rossiter, Grad Cert PTT, HScD, M N (NP), M Couns, B Couns, B Hlth Sc, RN, is a program convenor and a senior lecturer in the School of Nursing and Midwifery, University of Newcastle, Australia. She is a nurse practitioner in mental health and has provided therapy for many years. In addition, she holds a Doctor of Health Science degree.

References

Anazor, D. (2012). Preparing nurse leaders for global health reforms. *Nursing Management, 19*(4), 26–28.

Carrier-Walker, L. (2011). Focussing on the well-being of health care workers in sub-Saharan Africa. *International Nursing Review, 58* (3), 273–274. doi: 10.1111/j.1466-7657.2011.00933.x.

Crutcher, B. (2007). Mentoring across cultures. *Education Digest, 73*(4), 21–25.

European Commission (2011). *Consolidated version of directive 2005/36/EC of 24.3.2011.* Retrieved from http://ec.europa.eu/internal_market/qualifications/policy_developments/legislation/index_en.htm

Jokelainen, M., Jammokeeah, D., Tossavainen, K., & Turunen, H. (2011). Building organizational capacity for effective mentorship of pre-registration nursing students during placement learning: Finnish and British mentors' conceptions. *International Journal of Nursing Practice, 17,* 509–517.

Kim, J. K. (2011). The politics of culture in multicultural Korea. *Journal of Ethnic and Migration Studies, 37,* 1583–1604. doi:10.1 080/1369183X.2011.613333.

McCloughen, A., O'Brien, L., & Jackson, D. (2009). Esteemed connection: Creating a mentoring relationship for nurse leadership. *Nursing Inquiry, 16*(4), 326–336.

Nichols, B., Davis, C., & Richardson, D. (2011). Chapter 5: An integrative review of global nursing workforce issues. In A. Debisette & J. Vessey (Eds.), *Annual review of nursing research, 28* (pp. 113–132). New York, NY: Springer.

Patel, V. M., Warren, O., Ahmed, K., Humphris, P., Abbasi, S., Ashrafian, H., ... Athanasiou, T. (2011). How can we build mentorship in surgeons in the future? *Australian and New Zealand Journal of Surgery, 81,* 418–424.

Vosit-Steller, J., Morse, A. B., & Mitrea, N. (2011). Evolution of an international collaboration: A unique experience across borders. *Clinical Journal of Oncology Nursing, 15*(5), 564–566. doi:10.1188/11.CJON.564-566.

Chapter 8

Closing Thoughts: Reflections on the Mentoring Continuum

Billye J. Brown and Sister Rosemary Donley

In this chapter, Billye J. Brown and Sister Rosemary Donley provide their personal reflections on mentoring. They both continue to make significant contributions to the profession of nursing as leaders and mentors and have served as past presidents of Sigma Theta Tau International (STTI). Both of these chapter authors served as formal and informal mentors for multiple individuals throughout their nursing careers, including authors Baxley and Bond.

Mentoring Interview with Billye J. Brown

Billye J. Brown was the first dean of the school of nursing at the University of Texas in Austin. She is a fellow in the American Academy of Nursing (AAN) and received its President's Award and has been recognized as a Living Legend. In her interview with Susan Baxley and Kristina Ibitayo (conducted October 30, 2012, in Austin, Texas), Brown shared her thoughts and ideas on mentoring. Questions appear in bold type.

What is your personal definition of mentoring?

Mentoring is the result of an individual assuming the role of "the authority," or more knowledgeable person about an issue than another, and being willing to share information with the less informed person. Usually the "other" is a student, or person younger than the mentor, although this is not always the case.

The protégé is a less experienced individual who wishes to work with a more experienced individual.

Parents are the first mentors.

I recommend a mentor spend time socially with the person before accepting a protégé. Then the mentoring process is decided depending on what the protégé wants to do later; otherwise the protégé wouldn't seek out a mentor. This helps select the perfect fit. We had an agreed-upon set of objectives for the protégés I mentored as a dean-in-training (DIT), and they attended my classes with me.

Mary Toll Wright [one of the six founders of Sigma Theta Tau International] was one of the most important mentors in my life. I met her in Little Rock, Arkansas. She was my role model, as the word "mentor" was not used at that time. She was an important part of my life before I knew it was going to be important.

The term "life-coach" seems more prescribed. I had two protégés in a DIT mentoring relationship. One protégé was a Korean who studied the curriculum for 6 months and then returned to Korea and became a dean. Another protégé was a foreign student from Taiwan in a doctoral program whom I mentored informally.

Two other persons spent 1 year with me in a postdoctoral mentoring relationship. Each of them had objectives for their experience, and we reviewed the objectives to determine that their objectives for the experience were met.

When mentoring, are these mentoring components (challenge, mutually beneficial, respect, trust, communication, and cultural influences) a part of your mentor-protégé relationship?

Always.

Trust is the most important mentoring component. All I need to do is simply act my life. That's how you gain trust.

For formal mentoring, I had my protégés write objectives, as I wanted to see if I was able to meet their needs and if I was in a position to meet their objectives. That is why I agreed to be a mentor for both my protégés, as both wanted increased communication and political experience, although as individuals they were not in politics.

I had a weekly individual conference with each protégé over a 1-year period. This included planning for the next week. We would have conversations in the early morning, as both protégés were busy.

As a teacher, I always tried to share everything I knew.

What are some of the key factors that occurred during the mentor-protégé relationship (i.e., emotional support, knowledge, role-modeling, etc.)?

One negative result of the mentor-protégé relationship, which can occur and must be avoided, as it will interfere with a positive experience, is the development of a dependent relationship. This is not within the context of mentoring and occurs when protégés don't want to move on and want to ask what they should do all the time.

"The mentoring relationship is not at a mother-child level, but is at a professional level," I told my protégés. "I am not responsible for your decisions, but I am here if you need to call."

Which mentoring structures have you used (formal, informal, cascade, co-mentoring, e-mentoring, or coaching), and did these structures change over time?

I have engaged in different forms of mentoring (structures). In two situations, individuals petitioned me to mentor them, and I requested a formal petition which would outline their goals and expectations. In both instances, the protégé-mentee arranged to work with me over a period of a year. We had formal discussions of their progress at scheduled times during the year.

How do you think the process of mentoring contributes to the science of nursing?

When we determined that serving as a mentor was not a byproduct of nursing but an important part of the learning process of the professional, we were able to direct it to being both an art and a science. Research by several on the topic of mentor-protégé has helped develop the practice of mentoring.

STTI played an important part in my mentoring. After I retired as a dean, I became president of STTI starting in November 1989 for a 2-year period. I wish I had had experience prior to becoming a dean and help with leadership development. The idea for the leadership program at STTI was developed during my presidency, but I do not take credit for the idea.

What kind of expectations do you put on yourself as a mentor?

I would expect to set aside time to spend with the protégé and at scheduled times assess the progress of the goals, which would have been set before the agreement for the mentor-protégé relationship. I also felt in classes I taught that I was a mentor. I was also a mentor as a dean. I would:

- Facilitate the leadership development of the protégés and give them direction as they work to accomplish their leadership plan.

- Be a trusted and experienced guide. Be a teacher.

- Be a sponsor and supporter for future development of the protégé and a guide for professional goals.

- Reinforce positive qualities and work with the protégé to help develop qualities of leadership and mentorship qualities. Help with goal setting.

- "Be careful what you say, as you speak with great authority." A colleague shared this key tip with me early on in my role as a dean, and this was important in this position.

Which guidelines and expectations would you give a new protégé?

The protégé needs to "listen and weigh," not without consideration of his or her own goals and values. I was a protégé of the dean of the medical school in Galveston. The nuggets of wisdom I received from Dr. Truslow were on how to become an administrator: "Start thinking like an administrator."

What are the differences in mentoring BSN students, MSN students, and doctoral students?

One can expect a different level of maturity and a different set of expectations of students at each level. Examples of these are that:

- RN-BSN students are more socially advanced, because they have usually been through an ADN or diploma program and have developed social skills.
- BSN students think they have everything needed.
- Graduate students have mobility. They have developed their goals, whereas undergraduate students need assistance in setting their goals.
- For MSN students, you are "bringing them up" socially and academically if they are not already there.
- Doctoral students need to do several things before starting. They need to make sure their marriage is on track, have been to the dentist, had a medical checkup, and car checkup, as they won't have time once they begin the program. Mentors need to work with doctoral students as peers who have something to learn from you.

If you identify a need, suggest a solution, but it is up to protégés to decide if they want to do that. Mentoring is more personal, not being ascribed to each profession. You would use the same characteristics no matter who you are mentoring in whatever profession.

Which tips would you give both mentors and protégés?

Consider the responsibility that both persons must invest in a mentor-protégé partnership as well as the effort and time, personally and physically. Examine your current personal and professional situation and determine if the time and emotions invested in this role is advisable for you and the protégé.

Don't start a mentoring relationship without considering that it will take time and emotion. As a mentor, you are acting it out as much as verbalizing. In the DIT program, the protégés took on the aura of a leader unintentionally, such as how to dress and act.

As mentors, we need to be careful of the things we say to people. For example, I received an award for leadership at graduation from diploma school, which put the thought in my mind that I could be a leader.

Mentoring is a deliberate process, but the most successful mentoring does not appear to be deliberate. It becomes more inclusive rather than a list (i.e., when you ask for a list of objectives). The mentoring process evolves and is progressive, depending on the protégé.

In general, how did you assist protégés with negotiating the system?

Mentors cause them to examine their career goals and base their decision to join the venture with an expected outcome in mind.

When faculty members moved from one role to another (i.e., tenure-track to tenured positions), program to program (BSN, RN to BSN, MSN, and PhD), what challenges did you see, and how did you help them move into new roles?

I don't believe I did this as well as I would have toward the end of my tenure as dean. It is important to give people the tools for learning. That is what education is all about.

How did you assist those with different cultural traditions (by ethnicity), of different genders, and/or religions negotiate the system? (In general and in particular, persons of international origin.)

I have very little experience in this area, although two DIT protégés were from Korea and Taiwan, and I enjoyed my interactions with them. I respect others' belief systems and found it best not to discuss religion.

Brown summarized her thoughts on the interview and mentoring

Being interviewed for my thoughts about mentoring was a renewing experience for me. I have been a teacher for more than 60 years. During that significant largest portion of my life, it has always been important for me to be able to connect with my students, whether they are in the classroom, the hallway, or in a meeting room. I have taught all levels of nursing students, hospital diploma students and college freshmen through doctoral students. Each student has become an important individual to me. I needed to know them as individuals to fulfill my responsibility as a teacher. In doing this, I served as a mentor to each of them—not in a formal way, but always as a mentor. In retrospect, I believe to be a successful teacher one must also be a mentor. If this role became apparent to those students for whom I had the joy and privilege of serving as teacher, then I was a success as a teacher and a mentor. Mentoring should come naturally to the teacher. There was a time when I remembered the name of every student I taught—now that ability is fading, but with a little nudging, I will remember each one!

The following section contains Sister Donley's thoughts and personal reflections on mentoring. During her nursing career, Donley has served as president of Sigma Theta Tau International (STTI), president of the National League for Nursing (NLN), and the dean of nursing and later the executive vice president at The Catholic University of America. Donley is a fellow in the American Academy of Nursing (AAN) and currently holds the Jacques Laval Chair for justice for vulnerable populations at Duquesne University's School of Nursing where she teaches graduate seminars in health policy and social justice.

Sister Rosemary Donley's Reflections on Mentoring

Mentoring can be conceptualized along a continuum. On one end of the spectrum is the protégé; on the other, the mentor. These positions are not fixed; movement occurs along any continuum. As time passes, the distance between the protégé and the mentor is less evident as the protégé and the mentor move closer to each other. Often during mentoring relationships, especially ones that last over several years, the mentor learns from or is mentored by the protégé. If the mentoring experience is positive, protégés will be more likely to help and support others. Protégés become mentors.

In nursing, mentoring often begins in schools of nursing. Some students are mentored by their teachers, others by nurses in their clinical settings or student organizations. Kram (1983) describes the career functions that mentors perform for students and young colleagues. This is more likely to occur when the teacher (I am using the word "teacher" rather than "mentor") knows the students. Sometimes mentoring happens because a teacher recognizes a student's talent and potential. Often the student is not aware of his or her gifts. The teacher helps the student recognize and enhance his or her talent and flourish as a person and a professional nurse.

Some teachers think that mentoring is integral to the teaching role. These teachers make time to get to know their students, working with them in their development as professional nurses. Often mentoring is directed toward the perfecting of skills: writing, clinical, communication, academic, management, or interpersonal. Mentors encourage students to engage in volunteer and service learning activities and join and hold offices in professional student organizations, like the Student Nurses Association (SNA), their college's chapter of Sigma Theta Tau International, or organizations within the school of nursing or within the larger university. Faculty members also nominate and encourage students to apply for awards, scholarships, fellowships, or special activities. Interest in students' advancement extends the students' vision, enlarges horizons, and introduces the students to a world outside classroom or clinical walls. Mentoring facilitates maturation, self-esteem, and professionalism.

Not all mentoring is formal; sometimes the experience is subtle. It may be when graduates begin to practice that they realize that they have been mentored. Other teachers are more formal in their mentoring encounters. Usually these teachers discuss leadership qualities and personal and professional development experiences with their protégés. They identify opportunities; they engage protégés in new activities; and they coach, help, and encourage young nursing students to embrace the profession of nursing.

It has always interested me that nurses are recognized as being caring and very kind to their patients, but less tolerant of other nurses, especially young and inexperienced nurses. This dark side of nursing is told in stories about difficult and problematic relationships between teachers and students, staff nurses and new graduates, and old nurses and young nurses. It is also described in the literature (Dellasega, 2012; Ulrich, Buerhaus, Donelan, Norman, & Dittus, 2005). Some students see nursing school as a type of boot camp or a painful rite of passage. Others see their first job as the time in their lives that they want to forget (Morgan & Knox, 2006). Whether the old wives' tales are exaggerated or reflective of reality, focusing on intentionally helping young students or new graduates is a relatively new phenomenon in nursing. Mentoring has not always been a component of nursing practice or education.

Mentoring entered my vocabulary in the mid-1970s. I knew the word and had experienced mentoring by teachers, staff nurses, members of my religious community who were very experienced nurses, and others whom I met in my work and in civic and professional organizations. I thought of these persons who helped me as "special teachers," caring nurses or friends. I learned about mentoring in nursing from the work of another nurse, Connie Vance. Vance was then a student at Teachers College, Columbia, and was writing a dissertation on mentoring in nursing (Mancino, 2007). Lucie Kelly, my long-term mentor, was very excited about Vance's work, and she began to talk at the Sigma Theta Tau International's board meetings about the importance of mentoring. She saw mentoring as a responsibility of members of Sigma Theta Tau International. Interestingly, like "mentor," the name "Sigma Theta Tau" has its roots in ancient Greece. In Homer's *Odyssey*, Odysseus entrusted his property, but most importantly the care and education of his son, Telemachus, to his friend, Mentor, when he left his home to lead the siege of Troy. It was Mentor who led Telemachus in a search for his father. During the journey, Telemachus found not only his father but his own identity.

In 2007, Diane Mancino, the executive director of the National Student Nurses Association and a Teachers College alumna, interviewed Vance about her interest in mentoring. During her doctoral study, Vance had searched the literature on leadership behavior; she found that the term mentorship was "conspicuously absent from nursing's lexicon" (Mancino, 2007, p. 1). Vance found that nurses talked about "role models" or "preceptors," while other professions, notably business, used the term "mentor." Vance believed that although the term "mentor" was not found in the nursing leadership literature, nurses did mentor other nurses. In 1997, Vance wrote *A Group Profile of Contemporary Influentials in American Nursing*, in which she described her subjects' mentoring activities: "career advice, guidance, and promotion; professional inspiration and role modeling; intellectual and scholarly stimulation; teaching; networking and 'door opening' activities" (Mancino, 2007, p.1). Vance describes her work as the first study to explore the mentorship concept in nursing.

Kelly was a thought leader at Sigma Theta Tau International. She promoted Vance's work and created a niche as well as an award within the organizational structure of Sigma Theta Tau International to foster, encourage, recognize, and reward mentoring in nursing.

Today, Sigma Theta Tau International links the concept of mentoring to leadership development. Nurses and members of the society can participate in a wide range of mentoring activities to prepare them for leadership roles in academia and in professional, civic, and health care systems (www.nursingsociety.org/LeadershipInstitute). The mentors described by Vance shared a common vision: to formally and intentionally educate, guide, and direct nurses as they entered and advanced in nursing or changed career pathways within the profession.

This description of Sigma Theta Tau International's embracing the concept of mentorship does not convey ownership of the concept or a monopoly on mentoring activities. Today, most organizations provide formal and informal mentoring opportunities to their members, such as career-planning activities or helping nurses observe, learn, and then practice the skills and behaviors required in positions with higher realms of responsibility and influence. Systematically climbing a professional or organizational career ladder is no longer the only pathway to positions of influence. On-the-job training has been replaced with formal education, internships, residencies, fellowships, and mentoring. Other organizations offer guidance with particular skill sets such as publishing or grant writing; some groups assign their members to experienced nurses and administrators. Increasingly, foundations are requiring candidates for fellowships to find one or several mentors to assist them in navigating the cultures of research, academia, and health care services. Succession planning is a recognized management tool; contemporary leaders in health care and nursing are urged or required to prepare their successors. Although mentoring is now a recognized behavior of nursing's elite, Sigma Theta Tau International can take pride in being among the first of the nursing organizations to challenge its members to become mentors to the next generation of nurse leaders.

During her 2007 interview, Vance recalled that she had trouble locating the word "mentoring" in nursing's literature on leadership (Mancino, 2007). A recent online search of "mentoring in nursing" in *PubMed* yielded 2,915 references. The most recent article was published in the *Journal of Nursing Management* in May 2012; the earliest article was published in *Canadian Nurse* in August 1960. Articles on mentoring in nursing appear in international and national journals; titles listed in *PubMed* include descriptions of mentoring in acute care, workforce development, career progression, research competence, academic retention, and transitions into nursing practice (Byrne & Keefe, 2004).

I came of age when mentoring was an active process in nursing. The director of my diploma school emphasized the importance of joining professional organizations, especially the American Nurses Association and the National League for Nursing. I was convinced that membership in these organizations was as essential to practice as professional licensure. Several years later, the president of the Pennsylvania Nurses Association (PNA), my teacher in graduate school, appointed me to the Education Committee of the Pennsylvania Nurses Association. That year, the Education Committee was developing guidelines for awarding continuing education units to professional nurses. This experience was rewarding and instructive; it engaged me in nursing's collective effort to enhance quality of care and improve the educational competence of professional nurses. One day, I asked former teacher and PNA President Lucie Kelly why she nominated me to such an important committee; I was a young, inexperienced nurse and a new teacher. She said that I had written a very insightful paper on nursing education in her graduate class and that she thought that nurses in leadership positions should encourage young nurses by giving them professional opportunities. I had been mentored.

The literature has many definitions of mentoring. Traditionally, mentoring was defined using variables of age and experience. Like Mentor who helped Telemachus, mentors are usually older and more seasoned than protégés; they engage in relationships that help younger persons develop and mature personally and professionally (Kram, 1983; Levinson, 1978). Yoder (1990) notes that nursing's authors often use role-modeling, sponsorship, precepting, strategizing, and exchanging information as synonyms for mentoring relationships. She finds this lack of clarity to be confusing and not helpful to anyone who seeks to understand the mentoring process. The contemporary literature describes many models of how teachers nurture and prepare students and colleagues for outcome-oriented clinical practice, executive leadership roles, and academic and research careers. The literature also describes mentoring processes directed at developing workplace cultures that support professional human development, especially in acute care environments (Bally, 2007; Kelly & Ahern, 2008). Fagan and Fagan (1983) have found that mentoring increased staff nurses' job satisfaction. Other literature reports that mentoring is of value in retaining nurses in the profession and in organizations (Byrne & Keefe, 2004; Prevosto, 1998; VanOyen, 2005). Several themes are constant in mentoring definitions. A mentor is a wise and trusted teacher or counselor with something of value to offer a protégé. Mentorship is a partnership where sharing and growth occur in both mentor and protégé. Many articles identify outcomes of mentoring, including career development and progression, empowerment, social support, expanded knowledge, and professional socialization. There is another literature that describes the process, the "how" of mentoring.

Representative of the value that is given to mentoring in nursing communities around the world, Sedgwick and Harris (2012) describe a precepting and mentoring program that has become the cornerstone of clinical education in Canada. If Vance were a doctoral student today, she would have no trouble locating mentoring in nursing in the world's literature.

My mentoring experiences have been with academic colleagues and students; I advise and help them achieve their academic and professional goals. I listen and encourage them. I review their articles and reports, make suggestions to students and colleagues about dossiers or promotion papers, help with grant writing and research design, identify articles that may interest them, and alert them to other scholarly and professional opportunities that may be of interest to them. I recommend students and colleagues for honors, fellowships, and awards. I see these activities as preparing the next generation of leaders, expert teachers, and scholars.

What do I know about mentoring? Over the years, I have learned that nurses are not good at self-representation. They minimize their talents, accomplishments, and aspirations. Nurses find it difficult to convince deans, supervisors, colleagues, and foundation or grant officers that institutions or organizations should invest in them or their ideas.

Most nurses are not centered on themselves or their accomplishments. They are preoccupied with short-term goals, usually the desire to bring about some improvement for their patients, students, or other nurses. This desire focuses their attention on problems that affect individuals and centers their attention in immediate realities. Most young nurses do not use systems thinking or endeavor to bring about structural changes. Their energies are directed toward fixing current problems. However, the root causes of recurring problems and concerns in practice and education usually lie at the policy level; mentors can play an important role in helping their protégés expand their vision and orient their problem solving to system-level policies and processes.

Yoder (1990) finds that mentoring occurs in three forms: as a structural role, as an organizational phenomenon, and as an interpersonal relationship. In my experience, although mentoring begins because of the structural roles that mentors or protégés assume, mentoring in nursing is usually integrated into interpersonal relationships. Mentoring is not an integral component of the corporate cultures in most schools of nursing or nursing organizations. Because mentoring begins within the context of structural roles, most mentoring relationships are limited and temporary. Reflecting this observation, the nursing literature describes differences in short-term and long-term mentoring experiences (Eby, Durley, Evans, & Ragins, 2006).

What emerges as significant in analyses of types and expectations of mentoring relationships is that both mentors and protégés establish and honor the terms of the relationship. Mentoring is about trust. In any helping relationship, confidences are exchanged, and the parties in the relationship are bound to hold in confidence what they have learned and have experienced.

Like any relationship, mentoring has boundaries that must be respected. Establishing boundaries at the beginning of the relationship is important for both mentor and protégé. Most authors who write about mentoring discuss the emotional component of mentoring and the commitments that emotional relationships bring with them (Bowen, 1985). Although Bowen speaks primarily about the mentor, the protégé is also engaged in an emotional relationship. One pitfall to be avoided by the mentor is the desire to be overly helpful; help can become control.

Without intending harm, the mentor can take over the protégé's life and project her or his personal goals and aspirations onto the protégé. In my work in the social justice tradition, I realize that differences in real or perceived power can influence human relationships in positive and negative ways. Because power can be misused, abuse of power is frequently at the core of unjust actions, systems, and relationships. A mentor's possessiveness or control limits the freedom of the protégés and their ability to make their own choices about the future. One of the greatest gifts that a mentor can give a protégé is the freedom to make mistakes or even to fail. It is also possible for the protégé to become dependent on the mentor and become jealous of any attention or help that the mentor may give to another student or colleague.

Protégés also influence their mentors. They can teach their mentors about helping relationships in concrete, practical terms. Because the process of mentoring can be a life-changing event, mentors and protégés grow as the relationships mature and develop. Mentors can also experience satisfaction and rewards that do not usually happen in a class or a clinical unit. Over time, protégés and mentors can become friends and colleagues. Engaging in mentoring gives nurse leaders, teachers, clinicians, and scholars the opportunity to empower and emancipate members of the present generation of nurses and students of nursing. These experiences and opportunities contribute to the development of the profession. Mentoring builds a legacy that transcends individual experiences.

Conclusion

In this chapter both Brown and Donley commented on the mutual positive benefits when faculty members mentor nursing students. They indicated that the process of mentoring and the time span involved differs for each mentoring dyad. Brown recommends that prior to beginning a mentoring relationship the mentor and protégé meet socially, to see if the relationship is a good match and there are no personality clashes.

They both note that although the word "mentor" was not used initially in nursing, the mentoring process was still occurring. Donley notes that mentoring is needed since nurses tend to minimize their accomplishments and aspirations. Mentors may recognize hidden talents and skills in protégés and foster their professional and personal development. They believe that the mentoring process promotes individual development, and as protégés experience growth and become mentors in turn, the nursing profession is strengthened.

References

Bally, M. G. (2007). The role of nursing leadership in creating a mentoring culture in acute care environments. *Nursing Economics$*, *25*(3), 143–148. Retrieved from http://www. nursingeconomics.net/cgi-bin/WebObjects/NECJournal.woa

Bowen, D. (1985). Were men meant to mentor women? *Training and Developmental Journal*, *39*(1), 30–34. Retrieved from http://www. traininganddevelopmentjournal.com/

Byrne, M. W., & Keefe, M. R. (2004). Building research competence in nursing through mentoring. *Journal of Nursing Scholarship*, *34*(4), 391–396. doi:10.1111/1547-5069.2002.0039.x

Dellasega, C. (2012, January). Why nurses bully and what you can do about it. *Advance for Nurses*. Retrieved from http://nursing. advanceweb.com/Features/Articles/Why-Nurses-Bully-What-You-Can-Do-About-It.aspx

Eby, L. T., Durley, J. R., Evans, S. C., & Ragins, B. R. (2006). The relationship between short-term mentoring benefits and long-term mentor outcomes. *Journal of Vocational Behavior*, *69*(3), 424–444. doi:10.1016/j.jvb.2006.05.003

Fagan, M. M., & Fagan, P. D. (1983). Mentoring among nurses. *Nursing and Health Care*, *4*(2), 80–82.

Kelly, J. & Ahern, K. (2009). Preparing nurses for practice: A phenomenological study of the new graduate in Australia. *Journal of Clinical Nursing*, *18*(6), 910–918. doi:10.1111/j.1365-2702-2008.02308.x

Kram, K. E. (1983). Phases of the mentor relationship. *Academy of Management Journal*, *26*(4), 608–625. doi:10.2307/255910

Levinson, D. J. (1978). *The seasons of a man's life*. New York, NY: Knopf.

Mancino, D. (2007, Winter). Spotlight on Connie Vance. *Courier*, 1–2. Retrieved from http://www.tcneaa.org/images/Spring_07_Courier. pdf

Morgan, J., & Knox, J. (2006). Characteristics of best and worst clinical teachers as perceived by university nursing faculty and students. *Journal of Advanced Nursing, 12*(3), 331–337. doi:10.1111/j.1365-2648.1987.tb01339.x

Prevosto, P. E. (1998). *The effect of "mentored" relationships on satisfaction and intent to stay of company grade U.S. Army Reserve (USAR) nurses* (Strategy research project, U.S. Army War College, Carlisle Barracks, PA).

Sedgwick, M., & Harris, S. (2012). A critique of the undergraduate nursing preceptorship model. *Nursing Research and Practice, 2012.* 6 pages. doi:10:1155/2012/248356

Ulrich, B. T., Buerhaus, P., Donelan, K., Norman, L., & Dittus, R. (2005). How RNs view the work environment: Results of a national survey of registered nurses. *Journal of Nursing Administration, 35*(9), 389–396. http://dx.doi. org/10.1097/00005110-200509000-00008

VanOyen, M. (2005). The relationship between effective nurse managers and nursing retention. *Journal of Nursing Administration, 35*(7–8), 336–341. Retrieved from http://www. nursingcenter.com

Yoder, L. (1990). Mentoring: A concept analysis. *Nursing Administration Quarterly, 15*(1), 9–19. doi.10.1097% 2F00006216-199001510-00005

Epilogue
The Global Mentoring Process Revisited

Susan M. Baxley, Kristina S. Ibitayo, and Mary Lou Bond

The ideas contained in the chapters of this book and various authors' personal reflections confirm that the essential components and key factors of the Global Mentoring Process Model (see Figure 1.1, p.3) are indeed elements of the mentoring process and mentoring traditions. The concepts of "trust" and "mutually beneficial" were the essential components most often presented by chapter authors when describing mentoring. Other concepts frequently cited by chapter authors were support, knowledge, respect, and communication. Mentoring fosters development in the personal and professional aspects of our daily lives. Meaningful mentoring relationships are important, as they assist nurse scientists with fulfilling their potential and contributing to the science of nursing.

The globalization of health care and its related socialization aspects influence mentoring relationships. In less industrialized nations, Internet technology may be limited, necessitating more of a face-to-face mentoring relationship versus e-mentoring. However, nursing professionals seeking advanced degrees may rely on e-mentoring to access a mentor with similar research interests who may not be available locally. Another way to meet the mentoring needs of nursing professionals in less industrialized countries is by collaborating with nurse experts in other countries. Nurse experts can travel to these countries and conduct specifically requested workshops that meet local nursing needs.

The exemplars in Table E.1 represent the chapter authors' ideas of how they perceived Baxley and Ibitayo's Global Mentoring Process Model. The model's essential components (communication, challenge, mutually beneficial, respect, trust, and cultural influences) are necessary for establishing and maintaining a mentoring relationship.

TABLE E.1 Essential Components

ESSENTIAL COMPONENTS	EXEMPLARS
Communication	Culturally diverse students may communicate or interpret communication differently.
	Mentoring may be done in person, by phone, or by email.
	Mentor can help international/ESL nurse faculty with communication nuances.
Challenge	Students face many challenges related to finances, technology, and lack of a supportive environment.
	Mentor provides support to protégé struggling with faculty role.
	Challenges to mentoring include a lack of mentoring training and lack of time in a busy work environment.
Mutually beneficial	Relationships build networks of reciprocal interaction.
	Mutually beneficial partnerships advance both partners' career objectives in their specific specialized areas of teaching, practice, and scholarship.
	Everyone in the organization benefits from mentoring.

ESSENTIAL COMPONENTS	EXEMPLARS
Respect	Mentoring relationships need to be based on mutual respect.
	Respect is valued and takes multiple forms, such as mutual respect and respect for protégés' uniqueness and culture.
Trust	Reputation building, information sharing, and improved understanding of information that result from social ties provide a foundation of trust.
	One strategy for mentors is to establish trusting and ethical relationships with protégés.
	Protégés can talk with trusted mentors about concerns regarding being placed in clinical environments where they are uncomfortable.
	Ideal mentors build trust.
Cultural influences	Lack of mentors as well as differing language and cultural views are challenges for international students.
	The culture of each health care organization influences the success of mentoring relationships.
	Mentors need to be nonjudgmental and aware of the cultural biases they possess and show respect for protégés' cultural backgrounds.

The Global Mentoring Process Model's key factors, as shown in Table E.2, are knowledge, personal/emotional support, advancement, expertise, protection, loyalty, prestige, and role-model. These key factors promote the mentoring relationship and benefit the science of nursing. The concepts of advancement, expertise, prestige, and loyalty as presented by chapter authors were associated more with the work environment and a career.

TABLE E.2 Key Factors

KEY FACTORS	EXEMPLARS
Knowledge	Formal and informal mentoring fosters professional growth and may be part of the educational structure.
	The mentor helps guide which knowledge/skills would be a good fit for specific committees.
	The mentor and the protégé need to be secure in their own knowledge. The mentor needs to validate a protégé's knowledge.
	The knowledge the mentor possesses is positive and should be shared with the protégé, but that same knowledge can create a power differential/paternalism.
Personal/ emotional support	Mentors can offer compassion by providing a supportive environment and asking reflective questions of the protégés so that they can develop their own solutions.
	Mentors provide constant support when protégés are overwhelmed.
	A protégé is supported in the environment when mentoring is supported.
Advancement	Using complexity theory, especially complex adaptive systems, increases the likelihood of achieving professional goals.
	A main goal of mentoring is achievement of academic and personal goals.
Expertise	Proximity to and interaction with experts build expertise.
	Protégés need to seek the expertise of different mentors if goals change or if the current mentor does not meet needs.
	Gender may influence perception of expertise.

KEY FACTORS	EXEMPLARS
Protection	Mentors provide protection and a buffer against discrimination.
	Tenure provides protection of academic freedom.
Loyalty	A mentor's professionalism and attitude enhance a protégé's commitment and loyalty to the organization.
	Loyalty occurs when both mentor and protégé trust each other and believe in the mentoring relationship.
Prestige	A protégé may obtain prestige when working with a mentor who is a recognized figure in the profession of nursing.
	Some protégés may bestow prestige on the mentors.
Role-model	Mentors serve as role models.
	Nurse leaders serve as role models by creating standards of excellence in nursing education, sharing these standards with peers, and serving as role models of these standards.
	Role-modeling improves job satisfaction as the protégé emulates the mentor and attempts to improve skills.

For nurses to become a major force in influencing the science of nursing, they must embrace the idea of globalization. As the world becomes more connected and physical distance becomes less of an issue due to globalization, nursing professionals need to meet the challenges of the world's health care needs by embracing mentoring relationships within complex systems. In Chapter 2, Burns suggests that "systems thinking helps an individual view the system from a broad perspective that includes seeing overall structures, patterns, cycles, and emergence rather than only specific, often disconnected, events." (p.16). Nurses must mentor and be mentored to influence the science of nursing. Mentoring relationships provide a meaningful structure for nurturing nurses and equip them with the attributes necessary to influence health care around the world.

The following poem provides our perspective on the mentoring process. We view mentoring as a continual process, and this poem emphasizes the key influences of mentoring and how mentoring relationships may change over time. Trust is a key element in the mentoring process and is valued by both the mentor and protégé. When a positive mentoring relationship is experienced, the protégé in turn mentors others.

Protégé's Time Map
Kristina S. Ibitayo, PhD, RN

Trust, the essential ingredient,
As I place my hands in yours,
Bound to you for however long
Our mentoring journey takes.

Time appeared linear
The day I embraced guidance,
Seeking spheres of knowledge
To augment my own.

For a space in time,
I, as protégé, followed your lead.
When time's rhythm dictated change,
A harmony of reciprocal exchanges,
I gently let go of your hands
To seek those of a new mentor.

I too opened my hands,
Accepting the gift of trust,
The day I became a mentor.

A protégé's time map varies,
Dictated by each journey.
A constant remains,
Time is circular.

Time encircles me,
I am protégé and mentor.
The protégé's life cycle, full circle.

Appendix
Selected Mentoring Resources

Selected by Mary Lou Bond

This appendix provides a list of national and international resources that are available on the websites below. Because the term "mentoring" has frequently been used interchangeably with other terms, such as "coach," "guide," "tutor," and "supporter," it is not intended as a comprehensive list of resources. Additionally, some of the resources selected are from outside the discipline of nursing, as mentoring is widely used in a variety of disciplines both nationally and globally. Concurrent with globalization, Hispanics have become the largest ethnic minority in the United States. Therefore, a selected number of resources from websites in Spanish have been included.

Resources Within the United States

American Association of Colleges of Nursing—Leadership Networks: www.aacn.nche.edu/networks/rln/home. This site gives a list of leadership networks; membership is required for access to site.

American Nurses Association: http://nursingworld.org/DocumentVault/ NewsAnnouncements/Resources-on-Mentoring.pdf. Resources on nursing provide a link to several mentoring programs in the United States.

The American Political Science Association—Mentoring resources: www. apsanet.org/content_6514.cfm. This site offers information for those seeking mentoring and mentors and information on mentoring new and junior faculty.

Emerging RN Leader—A leadership development blog: www. emergingrnleader.com/about-2. Leadership development information incorporates best practices and research from leadership work being done internationally.

Georgia Department of Human Resources, Division of Public Health, Office of Nursing: http://health.state.ga.us/pdfs/nursing/Mentoring_ Manual_2006.pdf. This mentoring program is for public health nurses.

Healthy Wisconsin Leadership Institute: http://hwli.org/leadership-library/ mentoring-resources. This mentoring guide from the Center for Health Leadership and Practice of the Public Health Institute contains informational webinars and other resources.

International Mentoring Association: http://mentoring-association.org. This is a "premier" source for mentoring and coaching throughout the world, offering theories and practical examples of "best practices" for effective mentoring in global communities.

MENTOR: www.mentoring.org. MENTOR is an organization that promotes and advocates mentoring and is a resource for mentors and mentoring worldwide. Website contains extensive resources and publications.

The Mentoring Institute of the University of New Mexico: http://mentor. unm.edu. This organization was established to instill, foster, and promote a mentoring culture at the University of New Mexico. It provides certification, training, and evaluation and consultation services and sponsors annual mentoring conferences.

National Mentoring Partnership: http://www.mentoring.org. U.S.-based organization provides general mentoring resources, with an emphasis on youth mentoring.

National League for Nursing: www.nln.org/aboutnln/PositionStatements/ mentoring_3_21_06.pdf. Position statement from NLN advocates the use of mentoring as a primary strategy to establish healthy work environments and promote career development.

Robert Wood Johnson Foundation—New Careers in Nursing: www. newcareersinnursing.org/resources/mentoring-toolkit-dissected. This 76-page mentoring tool kit includes multiple handouts.

Sigma Theta Tau International (STTI)

- STTI Coaching in Nursing Workbook and Test: http://www. nursingsociety.org/Education/Leadership/Pages/Leadership.aspx

- STTI Building Research Competence in Nursing Through Mentoring: http://www.nursingsociety.org/Education/Professional Development/Pages/Professionaldevelopment.aspx

- STTI Mentoring Resources: http://www.nursingsociety.org/ Career/CareerMap/Pages/cm_mentoring.aspx

Transcultural CARE Associates: http://www.transculturalcare.net/cultural-mentoring.htm. This site offers tips for culture-specific mentoring and retention of minority students.

U.S. Department of Health and Human Services, National Institutes of Health, Office of Research on Women's Health (ORWH): http://orwh. od.nih.gov/career/mentoringresources.asp. This organization provides multiple resources, including guides for mentors and protégés, career development programs, and links to other resources.

U.S. Department of Personnel Management: http://www.opm.gov/ hrd/lead/BestPractices-Mentoring.pdf. This document provides information on mentoring best practices for both mentors and protégés, information on how to develop and implement mentoring programs, and an extensive list of resources and references that have proven successful in the field.

U.S. Department of Veterans Affairs: http://www.va.gov/nursing/docs/ research/nr_toolkit_www.html. This is a Veterans Affairs Nurse Scientist tool kit on mentoring.

University of Illinois at Chicago Mentoring Resource Guide: www.uic. edu/depts/hr/mycareer/images/uic_mentoring_guide.pdf. This guide outlines the benefits of mentoring for mentor and protégé, how to handle difficult situations, ways in which mentoring practices can improve, and a generous list of resources in the bibliography.

University of Washington: The Graduate school

- Mentoring Resources: http://grad.washington.edu/mentoring

- How to Obtain the Mentoring You Need: http://grad.washing-ton.edu/mentoring/students/index.shtml

- A Guide for Faculty: http://grad.washington.edu/mentoring/faculty/index.shtml

International Mentoring Resources
Australia

Australia Mentor Centre: http://www.australianmentorcentre.com.au. This site offers mentoring education videos with Australian thought leaders and fact sheets on topics to support mentoring.

Australian Apprenticeships Mentoring: www.australianapprenticeships. gov.au/program/australian-apprenticships-mentoring-package. The Australian Apprenticeships Mentoring Program is a new program that supports targeted businesses/industries (health care included) via mentorship and addresses workforce development skills.

Canada

Association of Public Health Nursing Management (ANDSOOHA): http://www.phred-redsp.on.ca/Docs/nursing_mentorship_resource_guide.pdf. This is an extensive resource guide for implementing nursing mentorship in public health units in Ontario, offering basic information about the concept of mentoring and processes for implementation.

Cancer Care Ontario—Palliative Care and Collaborative Practice Mentorship Program: https://www.cancercare.on.ca/about/programs/otherinitiatives/palcare. This site includes a description of the Palliative Care and Collaborative Practice Mentorship Program. This mentoring program in Ontario seeks to build supportive relationships between primary health care teams (protégés) and palliative care experts to increase collaboration.

Europe

BPW Europe Mentoring Program—Young BPW international: http://youngbpwinternational.files.wordpress.com/2012/06/bpw-europe-mentoring-program.pdf. The aim of BPW is to contribute to society by enabling women to sustain themselves.

European Mentoring and Coaching Council (EMCC): http://www.emccouncil.org. EMCC's vision is to become the go-to body for mentoring and coaching.

Establishing Mentoring in Europe: http://eument-net.eu/Documents/eumentnetManualWeb.pdf. This site offers strategies for the promotion of female academics and researchers via a guideline manual.

The Mentor Foundation—Mentor Sweden Projects: http://www.mentorfoundation.org/projects.php?nav=2-6-16. This site describes the need for adult role models among young people in Sweden.

Nursing Times: http://www.nursingtimes.net/opinion/book-club/successful-mentoring-in-nursing/5046994.blog#. This blog describes successful mentoring in nursing.

Japan

Mentoring in Japanese Nursing Education Community: http://www.sciencedirect.com/science/article/pii/S1976131709600190. This research study investigates the characteristics of mentorship in the Japanese nursing education community.

Russia

Role of Mentoring in Performance of Russian Women Entrepreneurs: http://www.european-microfinance.org/data/file/USASBE_Mentoing_women_entrepreneurs_Russia. Mentoring results are described in a sample of 500 women entrepreneurs in Russia.

Mentoring Resources in Spanish

Asociación de Enfermeria de Valencia: http://asoenfermeria.com. Tutoring is available for courses online. Tutoring contact (in Spanish) at tutorias@asoenfermeria.com. Nursing Association with 18,000 members in Valencia, Spain. Offers information, orientation, and documentation on employment, education, and training and works closely with the Valencian International University, offering courses online.

Asociación de Enfermeria Comunitaria, España (Congreso Nacional de Tutores y Residentes): http://enfermeriacomunitaria.org/web/ridec.html. Entrance portal to nursing practices in Spain. To contact, mail to presidencia@enfermeriacomunitaria.org. Nursing association organizes mentoring encounters in Spain and publishes a nursing journal called Revista de los Especialistas en Enfermería Familiar y Comunitaria.

Bibliografia y guias de tutoria usadas en la Universidad Nacional Autonoma de Mexico: http://www.tutor.unam.mx/do_libros.html. This site provides resources and references on mentoring as well as an online mentoring course. Contact buzontutor@servidor.unam.mx. UNAM (National University of Mexico) offers an online workshop at http://www.tutor.unam.mx/ap_taller.html to spread mentoring practices.

Consejo Directivo de la Asociación de Escuelas y Facultades de Enfermeria: http://www.aladefe.org. This is the Latin American Association of Nursing Schools. Each country provides tutoring resources to a different extent. To contact the association, the directory is found at http://www.aladefe.org/index_files/consejo/composicion.htm?reload_coolmenus.

Colegio Nacional de Enfermeras: http://www.cnemex.org/Sitio/index. php. Individual mentoring. The National Nursing College in Mexico is the governing body for nursing practices in Mexico and offers diverse courses to registered nursing practitioners. To contact write to conalenf@yahoo.com.mx.

Guia del mentor MAITRE: http://www.amitie.it/maitre/file/handbook_esp. pdf. This guide focuses on individual mentoring. It is provided by Amitie, an organization providing advice to European governments to develop education strategies. Amitie's phone in Bologne is Tel. (+39)051-273-173

Guia del Tutor de Grado de Enfermeria Consejeria de Sanidad, Comunidad de Madrid: A document published by Agencia para la Formación, Investigación y Estudios Sanitarios de la Comunidad de Madrid Pedro Laín Entralgo (ALE), but absorbed by Dirección General de Investigación, Formación e Infraestructuras Sanitarias. To contact phone number is (91)720-09-13.

La Asociación Mexicana de Enfermería en Urgencias: http://www.ameu. org.mx. Individual mentoring in courses. Phone number to contact: (55) 6304 0852. This is the Mexican Association for ER Nurses.

Nursing School Program at Universidad de Navarra: http://www.unav. es/master/investigacion-enfermeria/recursos_aprendizaje_modulov. Individual mentoring in the Masters Program. Contact: Navidad Canga Armayor ncanga@unav.es. This is a graduate program with an individualized focus.

Programa de mentorias- tutorias, para enfermeras en la Universidad de Puerto Rico: http://www.upra.edu/enfermeria/mentorias.html. This is the institutional program specifically designed for nursing students. Phone number to contact: 787.815.0000 Ext. 3250, 3260.

Universidad de Queretaro, Mexico: http://www.uaq.mx/servicios/desacad/ tutorias. Contact: meta@uaq.mx. This is an institutional program set in the university that is specifically focused on mentoring.

Index